You Can Beat Prostate Cancer

... And You Don't Need Surgery to Do it

What Every Man and His Family Must Know
About Early Detection and Treatment

**This is the book the author wishes
had been available when he was
diagnosed with prostate cancer.**

By

Prostate Cancer Survivor

Robert J. Marckini

You Can Beat Prostate Cancer
And You Don't Need Surgery to Do It

By Robert J. Marckini

ISBN: 978-0-6151-4022-3

"As a prostate cancer survivor and former proton patient, I find Bob Marckini's book to be the best source of information available to men who are at risk of prostate cancer, or have been diagnosed with this disease. There are lots of books out there, but none like this one. It's a straight shooting, nuts and bolts guide for ensuring you are properly diagnosed and understand the risks and benefits of treatment alternatives."

~Ken Venturi, Golf Professional and TV Personality

~

"It is a pleasure for me to give my unqualified endorsement to this comprehensive and truly interesting story by Robert Marckini. It should be read by every man who is diagnosed with prostate cancer. Prostate cancer in the early stages is highly treatable and can be cured. I am a senior cancer research scientist, pathologist and academic physician who was diagnosed with prostate cancer in 2002 and was treated with proton beam therapy at Loma Linda Medical Center. Prior to treatment, I went through the same deductive reasoning that Mr. Marckini outlines in his book and came to the conclusion that proton therapy would be effective for my treatment. Mr. Marckini has written his book with candor, warmth, clarity and insight. It will be a great asset to patients diagnosed with prostate cancer and who are trying to decide on what type of treatment to choose. I highly recommend it to anyone who is diagnosed with prostate cancer."

~H. Terry Wepsic, M.D., Professor Emeritus of Pathology, University of California, Irvine, CA. Research Professor at Long Beach V.A. Healthcare System, Long Beach, CA

~

"If you are diagnosed with prostate cancer, this is the *one book* you must buy. It explains all your treatment options from the patient's point of view. When I was diagnosed with prostate cancer, I read dozens of books on treatment - this book is by far the best of all."

~John Raynolds, Wayzata, MN, Cancer Survivor and former CEO of Outward Bound USA

~

"A landmark of a book. A provocative, intricate and intelligent study of proton therapy. A book to be recommended!"

~Ambassador Joseph Verner Reed, Greenwich, CT, Under-Secretary General, United Nations

"Bob Marckini's book was not only a crucial information tool, but it also blended the right amount of humor, background and fact. The author was able to deal with the serious nature of this issue, while never losing perspective of the rest of our lives. This book does an outstanding job of anticipating the questions that I and all new patients want answered."

~Jack Holt, Marblehead, MA, former CEO ACNielsen

~

"Robert Marckini was told that he was an ideal candidate, even a "poster boy", for each of three standard prostate cancer treatments, depending on the specialist at hand. His account of the resulting quandary typifies the wit and wisdom that fill "You Can Beat Prostate Cancer!" a book that any new prostate cancer patient will profit from reading. His choice, proton beam therapy, an excellent method with a solid track record, has been short-changed in the past because of ignorance and provincialism. Marckini's efforts are fortunately helping to change this situation."

~Herbert A. Klein, M.D., Ph.D., Pittsburgh, PA, Clinical Professor of Radiology University of Pittsburgh School of Medicine

~

"You don't need to read dozens of books, search the Internet, or interview hundreds of doctors and former patients. Bob Marckini has done it for you. If you have prostate cancer and are scared and confused, this is the book for you. I am a ten-year prostate cancer survivor. My experiences are comparable to those described by Marckini. I became frustrated and exhausted after hearing conflicting opinions from many different sources. Bob is an engineer with a brilliant scientific mind, which motivates him to investigate and understand how things work. This comes out in his book as he explains the details of each treatment alternative. Read this book. You'll need nothing else."

~Judge William M. Auslen, Carlsbad, CA

~

"This book, together with the author's website (www.protonbob.com), is a complete, user-friendly guide on what to do if you have prostate cancer, but want to avoid radical surgery. I am a satisfied Loma Linda cancer patient who struggled with what to do about it. I needed a book like this at that time, and we should thank Bob Marckini for filling that need."

~Doug Ayer, Greenwich, CT, Venture Capitalist

"Marckini has produced an exceptional work in sharing the trauma and the resulting journey associated with hearing the words, "you have cancer!" In a warm and convincing manner he conveys his personal search for a 21st Century non-invasive treatment modality for his disease. His journey ends in finding hope, healing, health, happiness and wholeness. It is a must read for anyone confronted with cancer."

> ~J. Lynn Martell, D.Min., Banning, CA, Special Assistant to the President of Loma Linda University and Medical Center

~

"I do not have prostate cancer, but I found this book to be a wonderful resource. Marckini's no-nonsense approach to health management was an eye opener for me. This book made me more aware of my responsibility for managing my own health."

> ~Edmund Butler, Mattapoisett, MA, Vice President (retired) Verizon, Corporation

~

"Do women have to worry about prostate cancer? Yes, they do! If there is a father, brother, husband, or a son, there may be a day where the issue of prostate cancer arises. This book should be of interest to anyone regardless of gender, who has been or will be touched by this disease. It provides the reader with a wonderful, thorough and compassionate orientation to find his or her way to the right decision for successful prostate cancer diagnosis and treatment."

> ~Arnd Hallmeyer, MD, Berlin, Germany, Prostate Cancer Survivor, pretreatment PSA 436

~

"Marckini has put together in this fine book the best of scholarship and deep concern for people. He writes with passion and the result is a book that should be in the hands of every man. I have two sons and will see to it that they have it. It is gratifying to see how proton therapy is making its way, sometimes against headwinds, toward full acceptance in the medical community. I was a member of the Loma Linda board when the decision was made to take the plunge, and now I am a graduate of the program. There was never any question about my going proton, and there could be no finer protagonist than Robert Marckini. I salute him. *He is a witness!*"

> ~Charles E. Bradford, President Retired The Seventh-day Adventist Church in North America

"Bob Marckini's book constitutes an important addition to the canon of literature on prostate cancer from the survivor's perspective. It is especially valuable to the individual who wants to avoid surgery. Bob covers his subject in a wonderfully comprehensive way. Style is direct and easy - - very accessible."

~Michael Keith, Boston, MA, Professor of Communication, Boston College, Author, Broadcast Radio Executive

~

"I found Loma Linda and Proton treatment by 'blind luck!' Bob removes the blinders and offers sound advice for those who hear the dreaded 'cancer' word."

~H. Jim Tuggey, Trophy Club, TX, Colonel, DMOR, U.S. Army Retired

~

"Already a leader in telling the world about proton therapy, Bob Marckini moves to the forefront with this intelligent book. Especially important to men wishing to avoid side effects of surgery and other forms of treatment. A must read for anyone diagnosed with prostate cancer.

~Bill Vancil, Media Executive, Madison, WI, Author of *Don't Fear the Big Dogs*

~

Adenocarcinoma – coming soon to a prostate gland near you! Now what? You could take the long, arduous, careful route taken by Robert Marckini in choosing a treatment – or, you could read his book. There is no other, single source offering a clear and concise route to the ultimate treatment decision.

~Roy Butler, PhD, Northfield, VT, Professor Organic Chemistry, Norwich University

~

"All men diagnosed with prostate cancer have options for treatment, and therefore a decision to make. The various treatments have been shown to offer virtually the same rate of cure, with differing nature and degree of collateral damage. Take your time, do your homework, and do *not* make your own decision without having read this valuable book."

~Earle Lipscomb, Sherman, CT, Airline Pilot

To my wife, Pauline
and our two children,
Susie and Debi,
for their love and support

This book is dedicated to
the extraordinary people at
Loma Linda University Medical Center.
They saved my life and preserved
the quality of my life; and for that,
I will be forever grateful.

Preface

My older brother had always been the strong one in the family. After my father died, Gene, then 45 became the patriarch. He took Dad's place as the family leader and he was good at it. Highly educated, well read, and in excellent physical condition, Gene, in his six foot one inch frame, became the one everybody turned to for advice and counsel.

Nineteen years later, in 1998 I was standing in the recovery room of a major Boston hospital when they wheeled Gene in from surgery. He had been diagnosed with prostate cancer three months earlier, and had undergone a radical prostatectomy (surgical removal of the prostate) on his physician's advice.

What I wasn't prepared for was how serious the surgery was, how deep the surgeon's scalpel had to cut, and how careful they had to be to spare critical nerves and blood vessels in order to give him the best chance of retaining his sexual potency and bladder control. I also hadn't realized how much blood he would lose – six pints in all.

There, lying on the hospital gurney was someone I barely recognized. His face was ashen; his eyes hollow. Attached to his body were numerous tubes, drains, IV's, a Foley catheter for urine drainage, an oxygen mask, and electronic monitors. My older brother, who four hours earlier was the picture of health, appeared to be inches away from death.

This experience had a profound impact on me. I had never seen my big brother in such a weakened and vulnerable condition. His situation was also of particular interest because my blood PSA was elevated and I was scheduled for a prostate biopsy the following week. Since both my father and brother were prostate cancer victims, my chances of being diagnosed with the same disease were high.

I made a promise to myself that day, that if I were diagnosed with prostate cancer I would do exhaustive research to determine if there were a reasonable alternative to surgery. Two years and three biopsies later, I was diagnosed, and I began my research.

I found four major treatment options for prostate cancer, and one essentially unknown alternative. The biggest surprise came when I discovered that the "unknown" option was quite authentic; it was painless; it involved no invasive surgery; and the success rate on thousands of patients treated over many years was comparable to "the gold standard," surgery. I also discovered that with this treatment there were minimal, if any, long-term side effects; and it was covered by Medicare and most private medical insurance providers. Yet most people, patients and doctors were not aware of its existence.

After completing my research, which included reading all available technical literature on and off the Web, and interviewing dozens of prostate cancer patients, I decided to have conformal proton beam therapy at Loma Linda University Medical Center in Loma Linda California. This decision changed my life.

The baby boomer generation is now approaching prostate cancer age, which begins in the late 40s and peaks in the 60s and 70s.

Most men will choose surgery for prostate removal on their urologist's recommendation. Yet most do not need a radical prostatectomy. They can be treated by other, non-invasive procedures, which provide comparable cure rates, carry far fewer risks than surgery, and preserve the quality of life.

One of these is a non-invasive, painless procedure known as proton therapy. The problem is very few people have even heard of this treatment. They soon will, as numerous medical centers all over the world are making the $100+ million capital investment in this extraordinary technology.

This book is my story. It takes you from the horror of being told I had prostate cancer through several anxious months of research, decision-making, treatment, and life after treatment.

This book is also a guide for newly diagnosed men and their families. It is intended to help them navigate through the myriad of technical details, treatment options, medical terminology, and the wide range of emotions that accompany this journey.

This is the book I wish had been available to me when I was diagnosed with prostate cancer on August 10, 2000.

Introduction

If you have recently been diagnosed with prostate cancer you are probably frightened. I was. You may also be confused. Most of us aren't prepared for this diagnosis. I had no symptoms. I was a physically fit 57 year-old non-smoker who ran three miles a day, ate a healthy diet and felt great.

And then the doctor told me I had prostate cancer. What do I do now? Do I put myself in my doctor's hands? Or, do I find out everything I can about this disease, evaluate *all* the options and make a decision that's best for me? Thank God I chose the latter option.

This is a true story of my diagnosis, my research into alternative treatments, my decision, and the outcome. It is also a summary of all the important things I learned along the way; things I didn't find in any of the books or articles I read about prostate cancer treatment; things I wish I had known from the start.

I make no claim that this is a complete and objective review of all prostate cancer treatment options. After hundreds of hours of research, I chose a relatively new approach called proton therapy. I admit I am now partial to this treatment modality. Why? Because it is non-invasive, it is painless, and it results in minimal to no side effects. But mostly . . . because it works.

I personally feel that anyone with early, mid, or advanced stage prostate cancer, without metastasis, should seriously consider this treatment, and I will explain why in this book. However, I must point out – I am not a doctor, I do not work in the medical field and what is presented in this book is purely my opinion. It is, however, an opinion based on considerable research, analysis, and interviews with hundreds of prostate cancer patients including many physician-patients.

This decision changed my life so dramatically that I feel compelled to tell the world my story. Whether or not you choose proton therapy as your prostate cancer treatment, you will find this book helpful in guiding you through the complexities of the journey you are about to begin.

Other Books on Prostate Cancer are Written by Doctors

In my research I discovered, not to my surprise, that the literally dozens of prostate cancer books available were authored by doctors. This, of course, gives the reader comfort in knowing that the claims made in the book are made by credentialed medical professionals. However, the books are often highly technical in nature and even with my engineering background, I had difficulty understanding some of the concepts presented. Also evident in my reading was the fact that each author seemed to "steer" the patient in the direction of his or her specialty. How objectively can a urologist – who is fundamentally a surgeon – write about radiation; a radiation oncologist write about surgery; or a brachytherapist write about cryoablation?

The question I kept asking myself was, "Whom can I go to, to find the best course of action for Bob Marckini?" After a while, the answer became very clear – *I* had to do the work; *I* had to provide the answers.

So, why should you pay any attention to a book written about prostate cancer treatment by a non-medical person? It's simple. Who better to tell you about such an important experience and decision-making process than one who has been on the receiving end; one who went through it himself? Who better can share with you the terror of hearing the news – "you have prostate cancer" – and then relate to you the story of how to deal with the emotions, the uncertainty, the ambiguity, and the unknown connected with understanding this dreaded disease, and then making life-changing decisions about treatment?

There have been literally hundreds of books published on the subject of prostate cancer and its treatment. Most of them are well written. They explain in great detail the technology and statistics from a medical professional's point of view. This book is intended to approach the subject of prostate cancer from the *patient's* point of view. Certainly any claims made in this book can be easily verified by talking with professionals in the field, by searching the Internet, or by talking with former patients.

As I look back on my hundreds of hours of research, the interviews I conducted, and the people I met during treatment, I am struck by the fact that the vast majority of men who elected proton therapy as their treatment option had several things in common. They were highly educated technical or analytical people who took charge of their treatment and were able to research, analyze, digest and understand the technical details connected with proton therapy. These men were doctors, lawyers, college professors, engineers, scientists, CEOs, physicists, and other professionals who were comfortable wallowing in technical detail and data.

But these are not the only kind of men who develop prostate cancer. What about the store clerks, policemen, postmen, janitors, plumbers, taxi drivers, and other men in our society who are not particularly technical or analytical by nature? What do they do when they are diagnosed with prostate cancer?

I found that most men simply put their treatment decision in the hands of their local doctors. While this may not be the *worst* thing to do, it was not for me. And, I learned in my journey that in many cases, turning this decision over to your primary care physician or your urologist is not in your best interest.

The deeper I dug into the various treatment options, the more I realized how important it was for me to take charge of my own treatment decision. In my research, I found that treating prostate cancer is not like fixing a broken bone, stitching a cut, or by-passing a clogged artery. There the choices are clear. With prostate cancer a patient's options are many, and they are diverse. How does one navigate through these alternatives and make an intelligent choice?

A word about How to Use This Book

This book is written for men and women. Women often play a key role in the research and decision making process for their loved ones. You will also find the book written in laymen's language. Highly technical terminology and jargon are avoided as much as possible.

In reviewing prostate cancer treatment options for example, I have attempted to cover the most important points in summary form and without technical details. Excellent resources (books, Internet, etc.) with significant detail are available to the reader for a more in-depth treatment of these subjects. Many of them are references for this work and are listed in the appendix. I have found that most people are not interested in the technical details, just the cold, hard facts.

Information presented here will be helpful to men who have recently been diagnosed with prostate cancer, men who have rising

PSA, and men who are at higher risk for prostate cancer due to family history. Men already treated for prostate cancer, who are experiencing a recurrence of their symptoms, will also find this book useful.

This book is also written for healthy men, those who take their health seriously, are proactive in managing their wellness, and are not waiting for the classical mid-to-late-stage physical symptoms of prostate cancer to show up before taking action.

You can either read this book front to back, or read selected chapters for information or to answer specific questions. Chapters can be read out of order and still provide continuity and value to the reader.

Helpful hints are found throughout the book as a way of highlighting key points. They are shown in bold print and italics for emphasis.

Readers often pay little or no attention to the Appendix in books. There is much valuable information presented in the Appendix to this book, and I encourage you to spend some time there.

Name Changes

Some of the names used in the book were changed to protect the individual's privacy. The people and situations described are all real, however.

Two Most Important Messages

Numerous points are made throughout this book that, hopefully, will aid you in your effort to prevent, cure, or otherwise deal with prostate cancer.

The two most important messages I hope you get from this book are 1) early detection greatly improves your chance for a cure, and 2) you can and should take control of your treatment decision. If you get nothing more out of this book than a clearer understanding of these key points, your time and money will have been well spent.

NO MEDICAL ADVICE: Material appearing here represents opinions offered by non-medically-trained laypersons. Comments shown here should NEVER be interpreted as specific medical advice and must be used only as background information when consulting with a qualified medical professional.

CONTENTS

APPENDIX

CHAPTER 1

Prostate Cancer – The Basics

"You will hear a lot of men who have been diagnosed with prostate cancer say they never had a symptom, never felt anything. That's because the most common symptom is no symptom at all." -- *Sidney Poitier*

Prostate Cancer is on the Rise

All forms of cancer are on the rise. According to Karol Sikora, former chief of the World Health Organization Cancer Program, cancer rates are predicted to double over the next 20 years. The number of new cases of cancer is expected to increase from 10 million per year to 20 million per year, and the number of deaths will increase from 6 million to 12 million.

What do we know about prostate cancer? We know that every 14 minutes a man dies of prostate cancer in the U.S. If you know a dozen men, two of them will be diagnosed with prostate cancer in their lifetime. More than 200,000 cases will be diagnosed in the United States this year. The prostate cancer diagnosis rate is increasing 10% a year due to increased awareness and improved diagnostic techniques. Prostate cancer is the second leading cause of cancer death for men, second only to lung cancer. According to the Cancer Group Institute, prostate cancer kills about 30,000 to 40,000 men each year in the U.S. alone.

We know that prostate cancer has affected some notable people including Senators Robert Dole and Jesse Helms, Generals Norman Schwarzkopf and Colin Powell, Nelson Mandela, Jerry

Orbach, New York Mayor Rudi Giuliani, movie personalities Sidney Poitier and Charlton Heston, sports figures Ken Venturi, Arnold Palmer, and Joe Torre, to name a few.

We hear about these high profile men who have gone public with their diagnoses. But what about everyday men like your barber, your plumber, your minister or priest, the trash collector, the postman, your father-in-law, your brother, and yes – even you? All are at risk of being diagnosed with prostate cancer.

We know that if you are African American, North American, or Northwestern European, your prostate cancer risk is higher than for other groups. We also know that if one close relative has been diagnosed with prostate cancer, your chances double. They increase five-fold with two relatives, and with three relatives your chances of being diagnosed are 97%.

What can you do about all this? Can prostate cancer be prevented? How is prostate cancer diagnosed? If you have it, can it be cured? What about side effects and quality of life after treatment? What's the best treatment option? These questions will be answered in this book.

Prevention

Little is known about the causes of prostate cancer. We know that your chances of having prostate cancer are greater if your father or brother has had the disease. Recent studies have identified genes that seem to play a role in this arena. Short of choosing different relatives, there is nothing you can do about the heredity aspect.

Some studies indicate that diet is a contributing factor. Reports from Harvard University have shown that Western diets, including those with high levels of fat from red meat and whole dairy products, increase your risk. Higher than average intakes of sugar, alcohol or total calories are also attributed to increased risk. Affluent industrial societies that consume large amounts of refined flour also have higher prostate cancer incidence.

Other studies show that eating soy, certain vegetables, fish, cereals and other whole grain products seem to reduce the risk of prostate cancer. Fruits, nuts and seeds also appear to reduce the risk of prostate cancer, yet the reasons have not yet been determined. One study proposed the benefits come from higher levels of boron in these foods.

Investigators at the American Association of Cancer Researchers (AACR) recently reported that a natural substance found in common fruits and vegetables significantly reduced the production of a key protein in hormone-dependent forms of prostate cancer.

A recent study in Italy compared 10,149 patients who were diagnosed with cancer between 1983 and 1996, to 7,990 patients who were hospitalized for non-malignant diseases. The results showed significant evidence that the men who ate larger quantities of whole grain foods had a 20% *lower* risk of developing prostate cancer.

Vegetable fats may reduce risk. A Canadian study involving 1,025 men found that those who consumed the most vegetable fats were 60 to 67% less likely to develop prostate cancer. Cruciferous vegetables, such as broccoli, cabbage and Brussels sprouts seem to be particularly beneficial.

A Loma Linda University study linked higher levels of tomato consumption to protection against prostate cancer. Higher levels of lycopene in the blood are associated with lower prostate cancer rates. A Harvard University study identified tomatoes as one of the most "productive" vegetables you can have in your diet. This has been confirmed in other studies as well.

Lycopene, an antioxidant, is the substance that gives tomatoes their red color. Very simply, lycopene helps prevent cells in the body from "rusting." In doing so, lycopene blocks the uncontrolled multiplication of cancer cells. If you cannot eat at least ten tomato servings a week, preferably *cooked* tomatoes, you should consider taking lycopene capsule supplements.

Asians are less likely to develop prostate cancer than their Western counterparts. Some experts feel this is due to the Asian diet, which is high in soy products such as tofu, soy milk, and miso. Asians also drink large quantities of tea. One study raises the possibility that there are compounds in tea that fight prostate cancer.

Finally, vitamin D and selenium, in reasonable doses, have been shown to lower the likelihood of developing prostate cancer in some men.

Since my father had developed prostate cancer more than twenty years ago, I figured I needed all of these things. My diet was already healthy. Red meat was something I consumed about once a month. Fish and chicken (skin removed) were a regular part of my diet. My wife always served lots of fresh vegetables at mealtime. I used very little sugar and my alcohol consumption was moderate. Multiple vitamins and whole grain foods have been a part of my diet for years. I had done my homework, so lycopene, selenium, and higher doses of vitamin D were already a part of my morning vitamin ritual.

Except for choosing different parents, I feel I did almost everything possible to minimize my chances of getting this disease. Nevertheless, I developed prostate cancer, as did my older brother. I concluded that there must be something to this heredity thing!

Based on my research, and discussions with patients, physicians (internists, urologists and oncologists), and health educators, as we men get older we should be taking multi-vitamins daily, along with lycopene and possibly additional doses of vitamins D and E.

In summary, no one can say for sure what men can do to prevent prostate cancer. What *can* be said, however, is that something over which we have no control, heredity, plays a significant role. It can also be said that you may be able to reduce your chances of developing prostate cancer if you eat a diet low in animal fat, sugars, and alcohol, along with fish, fruits, vegetables, soy, whole grain foods, nuts, and certain supplements such as tomato lycopene, selenium, and vitamins D and E.

What is the Prostate?

The prostate is a walnut-sized gland located between the base of the penis and the bladder. The urethra, a tube that carries urine from the bladder to the penis, passes through the center of the prostate. The function of the prostate is to produce part of the fluid that makes up the semen. During the process of ejaculation, the prostate contracts and forces fluid into the urethra along with the seminal vesicles, which surround the prostate. Sperm ejected from the testes also enters the urethra and mixes with the seminal fluids during orgasm.

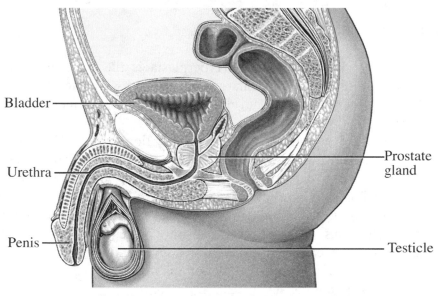

As men grow older, it is common for the prostate to enlarge. As the prostate enlarges there is a tendency for it to begin to restrict, or pinch-off, the urethra. This is a common cause of men's inability to completely empty the bladder. Unfortunately for many men, this creates the need to make frequent trips to the bathroom.

There are several diseases of the prostate. The three most common are prostatitis, BPH and prostate cancer.

Prostatitis

Prostatitis is a common infection of the prostate gland. The cause is not known. Some experts believe that prostatitis is an autoimmune problem. Others feel that prostatitis is a combination of several infections or diseases. Acute prostatitis with fever is usually caused by a bacterial infection. Yet other prostatitis symptoms have nothing to do with bacterial infection. Antibiotics are often prescribed for prostatitis and have proven to be effective.

BPH

BPH or Benign Prostatic Hyperplasia is the most common non-cancer cause of prostate enlargement in men. By age 60, fully half the male population will develop BPH. That number increases to 90% by age 86.

There are a number of treatment options for BPH. These include watchful waiting, medical therapy, balloon dilation, stents, and surgery. Every year in the U.S., approximately 300,000 surgeries are performed on men to relieve the symptoms of BPH.

The American Urological Association (AUA) has prepared a series of questions to help determine the presence of BPH. By answering these seven questions about the severity of symptoms, it is possible to define whether the symptoms are mild (0-7 points), moderate (8-19 points) or severe (20-35 points):

Questions to be answered: Over the past month . . .	Not at all	Less than 1 time in 5	Less than ½ the time	About ½ the time	More than ½ the time	Al-most always
1. How often have you had a sensation of not emptying your bladder completely after you finished urinating?	0	1	2	3	4	5
2. How often have you had to urinate again less than 2 hours after you finished urinating?	0	1	2	3	4	5
3. How often have you found you stopped and started again several times when you urinated?	0	1	2	3	4	5
4. How often have you found it difficult to postpone urination?	0	1	2	3	4	5
5. How often have you had a weak urinary stream?	0	1	2	3	4	5
6. How often have you had to push or strain to begin urination?	0	1	2	3	4	5
7. How many times did you most typically get up to urinate from the time you went to bed at night until the time you got up in the morning?	0	1	2	3	4	5

Sum of 7 circled numbers (AUA Symptom Score): _____

Prostate Cancer

Prostate cancer is clearly the most serious disease of the prostate. As mentioned earlier, it is the second leading cause of cancer death in men, surpassed only by lung cancer. Yet with early detection this disease is highly curable.

Prostate cancer develops from cells in the prostate gland. The most common cancer of the prostate is *adenocarcinoma*. Generally this cancer is slow growing. New detection techniques are allowing doctors to find it in the early stages. When this happens, the chances of a cure are very good. As men grow older and die of diseases other than prostate cancer, autopsies often reveal the presence of prostate cancer. It is often said that many men will not die *of* prostate cancer, but they will die *with* it.

Studies show that 92 percent of men diagnosed with prostate cancer survive at least 5 years, and 67% survive at least 10 years after treatment. If the cancer has not spread beyond the gland, the five year survival rate is 100% – again a good case for early detection. Unfortunately not all prostate cancers are detected early. According to a recent Harvard Medical School publication, when cancer has spread to tissues around the gland, as is the case about 31% of the time, the five-year survival rate is 94%. And for those men whose cancer has spread (metastasized) to other parts of the body – about 11% of the diagnosed cases – the five-year survival rate is only 31%.

Early Detection

Unfortunately the physical symptoms of prostate cancer often arrive after the cancer has had the opportunity to grow and spread beyond the prostate gland. This makes treatment more difficult, and therefore the success rate lower – all the more reason for routine testing to identify the presence of the disease at the earliest possible stage.

The importance of early detection cannot be overemphasized. Here is a summary of facts from the American Cancer Society and the National Prostate Cancer Coalition:

Approximate number of prostate-cancer deaths in U.S. in 2006	28,000
Approximate number of new cases each year	235,000
Lifetime risk of developing prostate cancer among American men (risk doubles if there is a family history of the disease)	1 in 6
Percentage of men who live at least five years after diagnosis	92%
Percentage of men who live at least 10 years after diagnosis	67%
Five-year survival rate for men whose cancer is confined to the prostate at diagnosis	100%
Five-year survival rate for men whose prostate cancer has spread to distant parts of the body at diagnosis	31%

I suspect that with improvements in detection and treatment in recent years, survival rates will continue to improve. And the value of early detection is obvious by these numbers. Early stage prostate cancer is almost always confined to the gland. Any legitimate prostate cancer treatment will destroy the cancer when it is confined to the gland. This last sentence bears repeating:

Any legitimate prostate cancer treatment will destroy cancer when it is confined to the gland.

All men should pay attention to the simple, low cost, painless tests that would virtually guarantee early detection, and therefore greatly increase chances for a complete cure.

PSA Test

PSA refers to Prostate Specific Antigen. This is a protein secreted by the prostate gland, which "leaks" into the bloodstream. A simple blood test measures the level of the protein in nanograms per milliliter. The normal range for a healthy man is reported to be between 0 and 4.0. If you have a PSA reading of 1.5, it means there are 1.5 nanograms (millionths of a gram) of the PSA protein, per milliliter (thousandth of a liter) of blood sample.

PSA levels between 4 and 10 are generally considered to be "borderline." Levels above 10 are considered to be "high."

The difficulty here is that PSA is not an *absolute* indicator of prostate cancer. A borderline or even high PSA is no guarantee that cancer is present. Similarly, a PSA result in the 0 to 4.0 range is no assurance that cancer is *not* present.

However, studies have shown that this important test is often a *relative* indicator of the presence of cancer and a red flag should be raised if the number is beyond the normal range, or if a rapid rise is observed *even within the normal range.*

PSA is also the key indicator of disease progression following treatment for prostate cancer (more on this in future chapters).

Any stimulation of the prostate can cause PSA to rise producing a "red flag" and needless worry. Digital rectal exam and ejaculation stimulate the prostate and should be avoided for two to three days prior to this blood test.

Digital Rectal Exam

The Digital Rectal Exam, or DRE, a simple, yet extremely important test is typically done by your internist during an annual physical exam. The doctor, wearing a rubber glove inserts his or her lubricated index finger into the anus and examines the prostate through the wall of the rectum.

A healthy prostate is generally small and supple. A diseased prostate can be enlarged with some indication of tumor presence. This can include abnormalities in texture, shape, or firmness. Often when a cancer has these characteristics, it has progressed beyond early stage.

Prostate cancer most frequently occurs near the periphery of the gland, so if a tumor is present, it can often be felt by DRE.

One limitation of this exam is that the finger can only reach, and therefore examine, the lateral and posterior (back) section of the prostate gland.

Most early stage prostate cancer patients have "normal feeling" prostates by DRE, and the cancer detection is done by means of a needle biopsy.

Transrectal Ultrasound

Another test used to determine abnormalities of the prostate is Transrectal Ultrasound or TRUS. In this examination, a small, lubricated probe is inserted into the rectum. High frequency sound waves emitted from the probe bounce off the prostate gland creating echoes, which are processed by computer and shown on a screen. Abnormalities not detectable by DRE can often be identified by TRUS. There is minimal discomfort and no pain associated with this simple and relatively quick test.

Biopsy

Typically your internist would refer you to a urologist when either your PSA is elevated or the DRE detects an abnormality. Your urologist would likely repeat the PSA blood test and the DRE. If either indicated the possibility of cancer, a biopsy would be ordered.

The prostate biopsy can be done one of three ways: transurethral (through the urethra), transrectal (through the rectum), or perineal (through the perineum, the space between the scrotum and the rectum). The transrectal biopsy is most common and will be explained here in more detail.

A probe is inserted to provide an image of the prostate. This image is used to guide the probe to the exact spot desired to remove a tissue sample. A hollow needle passes through the wall of the rectum, into the prostate and removes a core sample of tissue. This sample is packaged and labeled as to its location within the gland. Using this same technique, several more samples are taken from both lobes of the prostate and then sent to a pathology laboratory for examination.

If cancer is present, the pathology report will identify the specific type of cancer and the estimated percentage of the gland involved. The lab will also *grade* the cancer according to its level of aggressiveness. The grading system is referred to as the *Gleason* score. Lower Gleason scores generally indicate early stage, non-aggressive cancers. Higher Gleason numbers point to more potent malignancies.

Depending on several factors, a doctor may order additional tests to determine if the cancer has metastasized – spread beyond the prostate bed. For example, in the case of a borderline or high PSA, a palpable tumor by DRE and/or a moderate to high Gleason score, the doctor would likely order a bone scan, CT scan, or PET scan to look for the disease in other parts of the body.

Although not especially painful, the transrectal ultrasound guided needle biopsy is not an enjoyable experience. There can be some rectal discomfort for a few hours following the procedure, along with the presence of blood in the urine, stool, or ejaculate for several days to a few weeks.

Bone Scan

Bone Scan is a 2-Dimensional image of the skeleton using a radioactive tracer. This is a common test to detect cancer that has spread to the bone, a favorite site for prostate cancer to go to.

A scan of your skeleton helps determine if cancer has spread to the pelvis, lower spine, or other bone structures in the body.

CT Scan

Computerized Tomography (CT) is a 3-Dimensional image of the body using x-rays. CT is a commonly used 3-D imaging tool to help detect cancer that has metastasized (spread) beyond the tissue or organ where it started from. CT is useful when looking for the spread of cancer into the nearby bone and lymph nodes.

PET Scan

Most recently Positron Emission Tomography (PET) Scans have been performed to identify the presence of tumors. Radioactive glucose or other compounds are injected and tend to concentrate in tumor locations.

Chest X-Ray

Chest X-Ray (CXR) is a 2-Dimensional image of the lung, ribs, and back bone using x-rays. A CXR is commonly used to detect the spread of cancer to the chest area and for screening for other diseases.

MRI

Magnetic Resonance Imaging (MRI) is a 3-Dimensional image of the body using magnets and radio waves that is very different from a CT. Some of our tissues and organs are seen better by a CT, some by MRI and some by combining both. MRI is useful to detect the spread of cancer in the soft tissues.

Early Detection Summary

One of the most important messages of this book is that *early detection* greatly improves your chance of a cure. I cannot over emphasize the importance of early detection. If the cancer is identified before it spreads outside the gland the chances of a complete cure are virtually guaranteed. Also, by catching the cancer early, you have *all* the treatment options available to you. If, on the other hand, your cancer has spread to the margins, the seminal vesicles or the lymph nodes, treatment becomes increasingly more difficult, your options become more limited, and chances of a complete cure are diminished.

The most important thing a man can do to ensure early detection is to have annual physical examinations that include blood PSA measurement and DRE (digital rectal exam).

Other symptoms in the prostate region, such as urination difficulty, burning during urination, or pain in the pelvic region, should be called to the immediate attention of your internist or urologist.

Treatment Options

Once you have been diagnosed with prostate cancer the world doesn't come to an end. *Prostate cancer is not a death sentence.* In fact prostate cancer is not like many other cancers. Caught early it can be cured with a high degree of certainty. Even when diagnosed in mid and later stages it can often be effectively treated and cured.

When prostate cancer has been diagnosed, you fundamentally have six options available to you:

1. *Radical Prostatectomy*, or the surgical removal of the prostate

2. *External Beam Radiation Therapy (EBRT).* There are several forms of EBRT including:

   ➤ Conventional EBRT
   ➤ Conformal EBRT
   ➤ IMRT (Intensity Modulated Radiation Therapy)
   ➤ Proton Therapy

3. *Brachytherapy*, or radioactive seed implants

4. *Cryosurgery* – Liquid nitrogen freezing of the cancer

5. *Hormone Ablation Therapy (or Androgen Deprivation Therapy)* – The use of one or more hormones to shut down the production of male hormones, such as testosterone, that feed the cancer

6. *Watchful Waiting* (sometimes called *Active Surveillance*) – Essentially doing nothing except monitoring PSA over time, a perfectly viable option depending on circumstances. The New England Journal of Medicine recommends against Watchful Waiting if life expectancy is greater than five years

These alternatives are all discussed in some detail in later chapters.

A relatively new option, called HIFU, or High Intensity Focused Ultrasound, practiced in Europe and Canada is showing promise. But there is minimal data available on cure rates and side effects at this writing, so it will not be discussed here.

How Do You Know if You're Cured?

Once you have chosen one of the above treatment options, how do you know if it worked? There is disagreement in the medical community on this subject. Cancer is much different from other medical conditions. When a broken bone is repaired, you know it. When heart by-pass surgery is completed you know the restriction has been eliminated. When an infection has been destroyed, analytical measurements can confirm this.

But cancer is insidious, in that microscopic cells can linger close to the original cancer site, or can migrate through different channels to other parts of the body. There, they can establish colonies and continue their dirty work. For that reason cancer patients need to be monitored for some time to determine if the cancer has been completely removed or destroyed.

For prostate cancer patients, the best measure is PSA. PSA in the blood can only come from two places – a functioning prostate or prostate cancer cells. In the case of surgery, where the prostate is removed, a patient's PSA should drop to zero, or less than 0.1 ng/ml, the detectable limit. A result higher than that is an indication of prostate cancer – or laboratory error. The latter possibility is always reason to repeat the blood test and lab analysis.

When the prostate is left in place, as is the case for all other treatment options, there will usually be some PSA in the blood from a functioning, or even partially functioning prostate gland. But increasing levels of PSA are of concern. For this reason, PSA is still the primary measure of cancer activity, backed up with periodic digital rectal exams (DREs) – but PSA is treated differently in this case.

All forms of radiation as well as cryosurgery damage cancer cell DNA. This is covered in more detail in later chapters. Damaged DNA results in something called apoptosis, or programmed cell death, or in necrosis, another form of cell death. The damaged cancer cells will live for some time, but they cannot reproduce and therefore eventually die off.

For these patients, PSA is tracked periodically, usually every six months, for several years.

There are two terms used by physicians to report on success or failure of prostate cancer treatment: bNED and cNED.

bNED, refers to no *biochemical* evidence of disease. The American Society for Therapeutic Radiology and Oncology (ASTRO) considers one to be biochemically free of prostate cancer as long as the patient's PSA remains essentially flat after it reaches its low point, or nadir. If there are three successive rises in PSA of 10% or more, one *may* have experienced *biochemical* failure, i.e., prostate cancer may have returned. Several laboratory tests are available to determine if in fact this is the case.

The term cNED refers to no *clinical* evidence of disease. The clinical test for disease is the Digital Rectal Exam (DRE). If the physician notices a lump by DRE, in a patient where there was no prior lump; or if an existing lump (tumor) is growing larger, the patient may have experienced *clinical* failure. Before the PSA test was available, the DRE was the only test available to monitor progress following treatment for prostate cancer.

bNED and cNED are used in combination to monitor cure rates for prostate cancer patients. Generally speaking, the lower the nadir post treatment, the better are the chances of long term bNED and cNED (i.e., cure). Studies of radiation-treated patients typically compare patients with nadirs in three categories: 1) PSA less than 0.5, 2) 0.5 to 1.0 and, 3) greater than 1.0. The first category, less than 0.5 post treatment, is clearly the most desirable.

Become Your Own Advocate

This is perhaps the most important message of this book. *You need to take charge of your own treatment decision.* No single treatment is best for everybody. In the case of prostate cancer, you have several treatment alternatives, and there is only one person on this planet who is qualified to choose the option that is best for you. *You!* But you need to do your homework first, so that you are comfortable with your decision.

Most of us were brought up to believe the doctor knows best. One of the most common questions a prostate cancer patient asks his doctor is "What would you do if you were me, doctor?" And the doctor will tell you. But what you need to realize is that doctors in different specialties will often give you different answers to that question. Let me repeat this very important point:

Doctors in different specialties will often give you different answers to the question, "What would you do doc?" And most are biased to their specialty.

In the course of my interviews of hundreds of prostate cancer patients, the vast majority of them reported that when they met with their urologist, who is fundamentally a surgeon, surgery was recommended. The radiation oncologist typically recommended radiation. Those who met with doctors specializing in brachytherapy were generally encouraged to do seed implants. Cryo-surgeons recommended freezing, and so on. How can surgery, external beam radiation, seeds and liquid nitrogen all be *best* for the same patient? They can't.

Does this mean that doctors are intentionally misleading their patients for their own personal gain? No. Most doctors will act in terms of what they believe is in the best interest of their patients. Sadly, many doctors are not knowledgeable about some of the developing technologies. Therefore it is up to you, the patient, to do your own homework, and make the treatment decision that is best for *you.*

I happened to choose proton beam therapy (PBT, a form of external beam radiation) for my treatment. My own urologist, who is chief of urology for a major hospital in the Northeast, admitted lack of knowledge of proton beam treatment and encouraged me to have surgery. Why? Because he was very experienced, he had done several hundred surgeries, he believed that considering my age, physical condition, PSA, and Gleason score, surgery offered me the best chance for a cure.

The radiation oncologist, said, "Considering your age, cancer stage, and general health, I recommend Conformal External Beam Radiation Therapy."

The brachytherapist felt similarly about his specialty. He told me that I was "the poster boy for brachytherapy." Why? Because of my relatively young age, good health, non-enlarged prostate, early stage cancer, and his experience and expertise at his specialty.

The doctor I spoke with about cryosurgery felt the same way. If he were in my shoes he would choose to freeze the prostate.

How could each of these treatment options be best for me? I knew they couldn't. They might all have worked, but what about such issues as impotence, incontinence, fatigue, pain, convenience, cost, treatment time, recuperation time, and other factors that were important to me?

I quickly learned one of the most important lessons of this journey: *The only way I can know for sure what is best for me is to jump in with both feet, learn everything I can about each option and then make my own decision.* I did this, and my ultimate decision surprised everyone – especially me.

When I was first diagnosed with prostate cancer and did my preliminary research, proton beam therapy wasn't even on my radar screen. I didn't know it existed. I now head up an international support group for men who have chosen PBT. I therefore admit a built-in prejudice toward this option. But I do not think it is for everybody. And I truly believe that by reading and understanding what is presented in this book, you too will make the decision that is best for you.

Commonly Asked Questions

There are two questions men and their partners often think about and are afraid or embarrassed to ask. The first: "Is there any connection between the level of a man's sexual activity (i.e. the *use* of the prostate) and prostate cancer?" The answer is no. Although some have theorized that inactive prostates are more prone to cancer, both sexually active men and celibate men develop prostate cancer at about the same rate.

The second question: "If I am diagnosed with prostate cancer, can I give it to my wife when we have sex?" Again, the answer is no. Prostate cancer is not contagious or transmittable during intercourse.

Summary

You must take charge of your own case in order to make the best decision for *you*. Prostate cancer is different from other cancers, and prostate cancer treatment options are all very different from each other.

In the case of prostate cancer, *you* need to take control of the decision-making process. Doing so can make a world of difference in the success of your treatment and in the quality of your life following treatment. The remainder of this book is about what you need to do to take control of the detection and treatment of prostate cancer.

CHAPTER 2

My Early Indications of Prostate Cancer

"Nothing in life is to be feared, it is only to be understood."
– Marie Curie

Dad was First

I was a little boy when my father had his operation. Back then you didn't say the word "cancer" in our house. The word wasn't allowed in our vocabulary. Occasionally my mother would refer to the dreaded disease as "the big C."

My father's operation for prostate cancer was kept a secret from friends and family. Not even his four children were told why he was in the hospital. He was just having an operation on his "private parts."

He survived the operation and had no indications of cancer recurrence. Of course this was before PSA was measured, so we didn't know for sure if the cancer was still growing in his body. Years later, he also survived colon cancer– another secret that was kept from the children. And when he passed away in 1978, it was from a stroke – totally unrelated to his two encounters with "the big C." I later learned how important a role heredity plays in the cancer puzzle, and how much more vigilant my brother and I should have been.

The Early Signs were There

Physical fitness was always important to me. I always paid attention to my diet and began jogging for health in my early 30s. From that time forward, I ran and exercised 3 to 4 days a week.

Annual physicals were also a part of my regimen beginning at age 40. Before then my physicals were randomly spaced.

I monitored my blood pressure, cholesterol level, triglycerides and other factors. It wasn't until my early 50s that I started paying attention to my PSA.

Not much had been published about PSA in the 1970s and 80s. But its validity as a prostate cancer marker was becoming more and more widespread.

As far back as I can recall, my PSA was on the high side of "normal." The early measurements ranged from about 2.5 to 3.5. Nothing to be alarmed about – or so I was told. I didn't know then that I was at high risk, and perhaps should have been biopsied years earlier.

In my mid-50s, my PSA began to rise slowly, approaching 4.0.

My Brother's Turn

Coincidentally, Gene, my older brother by six years, had been experiencing a rise in his PSA. Routine DREs (digital rectal exams) did not detect any abnormalities in his prostate. However, when his PSA moved beyond the normal range, his urologist ordered a needle biopsy. The results came back positive for prostate cancer.

Gene then did what most of us would do. He consulted his urologist. "Go with the 'gold standard,' surgery," the doctor advised. Gene, a busy businessman, took that advice and his radical prostatectomy was set for one month later. This gave him time to 'bank' four pints of blood in the event he needed it during surgery. As it turned out, he needed six.

His wife, Toni, and I were with him just before surgery and I remember the worried look on his face. Gene, being justifiably frightened, always a bit melodramatic – and now in the role of the family patriarch – began lecturing me on my responsibilities. "If anything happens to me, Bob, you need to step into my role. Make sure mom is taken care of, help Toni handle my affairs, keep an eye on my kids, and stay close to your sisters." Until then, I had not given much thought to my brother's, or my own mortality. It was a sobering experience. I wasn't ready for – and I didn't want – the patriarch role.

They wheeled Gene in to surgery while Toni and I waited. I knew enough about the procedure to understand this was *major* surgery, and there were always chances of complications. So, we stayed at the hospital to await the outcome.

Four hours later it was over and he was brought in to the recovery room. Within minutes of his arrival, Toni and I were allowed to visit. We were told the operation went well, and that he was still groggy from the anesthesia. In retrospect, that visit had a monumental impact on me.

At first I didn't recognize him. He seemed to have shriveled in size. The tubes and wires attached to him intimidated me. It was hard to believe this was my big brother, the guy who always beat me at every game we played; the patriarch, the cornerstone of our family.

Tip: If you have decided on surgery as treatment for your prostate cancer, do not visit a friend or relative who has had this procedure for at least 24 hours after the operation. A visit soon after surgery may change your mind.

Tip: If you are looking for a reason to eliminate surgery as an option, visit someone who has had this procedure soon after the operation was completed.

I Could Be Next

It was then I realized I might be in for a similar fate, as my PSA was rising.

While in the recovery room with my brother, I decided that if I were ever diagnosed with prostate cancer, I would make every effort to find an alternative to surgery to avoid the trauma, blood loss, and side effects.

Radical prostatectomy just seemed too barbaric to me. Even the term "radical" instills fear. The prostate is located deep inside the torso; lots of "parts" need to be displaced to access this gland; it is surrounded by delicate organs that are critical to maintaining sexual function and bladder control; and the operation can be extremely bloody.

PSA Rising

My PSA continued to rise, and when it broke through the "magic" 4.0 and hit 4.2, my internist recommended I see a urologist.

The urologist conducted a DRE, which was normal. He next did an ultrasound, which indicated a normal sized prostate with no unusual characteristics. And finally, he took a blood sample for PSA. The lab results of the blood test confirmed the initial 4.2 reading. The urologist told me he wasn't particularly concerned, but suggested that I retest my PSA in six months.

I later learned that I was at high risk, and that a biopsy should have been ordered at that time, or even a year earlier, when my PSA had risen from 3.1 to 3.9.

The six-month PSA was 4.6. It was time for a needle biopsy.

My First Biopsy

This was an interesting experience, to say the least. First of all, I did not know there were different "techniques" involved in taking biopsy samples. Neither did I know that the number of biopsy samples taken varied from urologist to urologist, from 6 to 24. Nor did I know that I could have opted for local anesthesia to ease the pain and discomfort.

My urologist told me the biopsy would be quick and relatively painless; and though it might be a little uncomfortable, it would be over before I knew it. As it turned out, he was wrong on all counts. He informed me he was planning to insert an ultrasound tube in my rectum to produce an image of my prostate to help determine where to take samples. While the tube was inserted, he said he would insert another device, a spring-loaded hollow needle, which would pass through my rectal wall, into my prostate and remove samples for analysis.

I remember saying, "You mean to tell me that you're going to fire a dart through my rectum, and rip out a chunk of my prostate?" He said, "Well that's one way to put it." "How many times will you do this?" I wanted to know. "Six" he replied. "Are you sure it won't hurt?" I asked. "Well, it might hurt a little. But it'll be over before you know it." Wrong and wrong. It later occurred to me that he would have no way of knowing if it hurt or not. He had never been on the receiving end of this test!

The morning of the biopsy, I didn't have much of an appetite for breakfast. I had some juice and coffee, took the antibiotic prescribed to prevent infection, and drove to the urologist's office.

As directed, I removed my clothes, climbed up on the table and rolled over on my left side. I was feeling particularly vulnerable, knowing, I thought, what was to happen next.

This urologist worked alone, which I later discovered was a big disadvantage for me. He began by inserting a large diameter tube that felt like an aluminum baseball bat. Next came his vintage ultrasound probe. Then he inserted the spring-loaded needle. It felt as though everything on his shelf was being loaded into my rectal cavity. Next he fired the first shot. Snap! That's the sound you hear while you experience a strange sensation in your lower rectum, similar to an instantaneous, painful hemorrhoid.

Things began to get worse. Because he worked alone, he had no one to package and label the sample. So, he had to remove the needle, the ultrasound probe, the baseball bat, and the other paraphernalia.

After packaging and labeling the sample, he re-inserted the entire ensemble and repeated the procedure – five more times. This less-than-pleasant procedure took about 30 minutes. What happened to, "It'll be over before you know it?"

Tip: Before having a prostate biopsy, find out if your doctor does this procedure alone, or if he uses an assistant. If he works alone, find another urologist. This procedure can be completed in less than ten minutes with two people working together – one sampling, the other packaging and labeling.

I cannot say that the procedure was extremely painful. Some men claim it's a "piece of cake" (remind me to avoid their bakery). But for me, and others I have interviewed, it was quite uncomfortable. I was left with what can best be described as a "bad headache" in my rectum. After an over-the-counter pain-killer and a few hours of rest the pain was gone, but not the side effects. For about two weeks I had blood in my urine, ejaculate and stool. This is not uncommon following a prostate biopsy.

> *Tip: Some urologists use a local anesthetic to eliminate pain during prostate biopsy. Find a urologist who will do this. It will make all the difference in the world in your experience of this procedure.*

First Biopsy Results

This next part was difficult. My heart goes out to anyone who has ever had a biopsy – prostate or otherwise – the waiting is torture. A week went by and I called the doctor's office as requested. I braced myself for the worst and prayed for the best.

The doctor was not in, but his office manager told me she would look up the results. Her search took about three minutes, which felt like three hours. "Good news" she said. "The biopsy was negative."

I gasped as I let out the breath I had been inadvertently holding while waiting on the phone, and I thanked her profusely – as if she had something to do with the wonderful results.

Later the doctor called me and told me he wanted to see me again in one year.

My PSA Continues to Rise

A year later my PSA had risen to 5.2 and my urologist ordered another biopsy.

By this time I had done a little research. I had discovered that other urologists worked with biopsy sampling specialists using more modern and, thankfully, smaller equipment, and more streamlined techniques.

I decided to switch urologists and chose one who was a prominent physician in a well-known Boston hospital. His technique was no 'walk in the park,' but it was infinitely better than my previous doctor's procedure.

With coffee, juice and antibiotic in place I drove to the urologist's office, and, for some reason, I was less apprehensive than the first time I went through this routine.

I didn't have to remove my clothes, just climb up on the table, slide my pants and shorts below my knees and roll over on my left side. A much smaller broomstick-sized device was inserted in my now highly-explored rectum. The ultrasound probe and spring-loaded needle were inserted in tandem.

A sample was taken, "snap." Then another, "snap." And then four more, "snap, snap, snap, snap." The two men talked and joked during the procedure, which actually relaxed me. I found myself joining in the conversation and joking along with them. Five or six minutes later it was over. Having a two-man team permitted them to grab and package the samples without having to remove and reinsert the "broomstick," which made the entire ordeal much more tolerable and of significantly shorter duration. This pleased me to no end – pun intended. Yes, there was some pain, but less than before, and it was over so quickly, I didn't really have time to think about it.

Tip: Talk with others who have been biopsied. Find out if their doctors used the most modern equipment and procedure. Determine how long the procedure took and how much discomfort they experienced. A prostate biopsy does not have to be painful.

Despite the dramatically improved equipment and procedure, the side effects were the same. Soreness for several hours, plus blood in my urine, stool and ejaculate.

Second Biopsy Results

Another week of torture. This time I knew I would get the news while cruising the Atlantic with two friends. We were running a boat up to Massachusetts from South Florida. During the trip, I was a bit preoccupied with the news I would be receiving that week. I had a gnawing feeling the test results would be positive and I would be told I had prostate cancer. I kept picturing my brother in the recovery room. Then saw myself in his place with tubes, drains, catheters and such. Not a pretty picture.

We were off the coast of North Carolina when I called my doctor's office from the cell phone on the designated day. The receptionist put me in touch with a nurse who told me she couldn't lay her hands on my test results, and suggested that I call back in an hour – sixty more agonizing minutes.

I called back. This time she had the results, and again, good news, the biopsy was negative! I remember telling this woman that I loved her and I would be sending her flowers.

We had dinner that night on the boat, and I recall having an extra martini with my friends to celebrate the good news.

But I still had to face one indisputable fact. My PSA was rising, and that wasn't good.

CHAPTER 3

The Dreaded Diagnosis

*"When you get into a tight place and it seems that you can't go on,
hold on – for that's just the place and the time that the tide will turn."*
– Harriet Beecher Stowe

PSA Rises Further – and Now a *Free* PSA Signal

Six months later my PSA was 6.6 and six months after that, it had reached 7.5. To add to my fears, my doctor ordered a relatively new test called *Free* PSA. This is a test that measures the amount of unbound, or "free" prostate-specific antigen in the blood. It helps determine the degree to which high PSA may be related to cancer versus other benign conditions.

In my case both numbers were where they shouldn't be. PSA was now 7.9, and "Free PSA" was low at 7%, indicating a 56% probability that I had prostate cancer. Free PSA is discussed in another chapter.

It was time for another biopsy.

This time I went to the same urologist and he used the same technique – uncomfortable, but tolerable. And I had the same side effects.

Tip: If you have rapidly rising PSA, whether or not it is outside the normal range and whether or not you have an abnormal DRE, have your doctor instruct the laboratory to run a "Free PSA" test in addition to the standard PSA test. It costs a few dollars more and it takes a few more days to get the results, but this test can provide valuable data indicating the probability of prostate cancer, well before a biopsy is called for.

Third Biopsy Results – "The Big C"

It was August 2000. I was with my wife and a group of friends vacationing in Nantucket on my boat. Since I was expecting bad news this time, I told my doctor I would call him for the test results *after* I returned from vacation a week later – I really didn't want to know the results until I returned home.

Unfortunately, my doctor forgot my request. On Thursday, August 10, 2000 I decided to check my messages at home using my cell phone. There were five messages, one of which I remember clearly: "Mr. Marckini, this is Dr. Parker, I have your biopsy results and I'd like you and your wife to meet with me in my office this Friday. Please call for an appointment." Not the most sensitive way to deliver an obvious and ominous message.

This message could mean only one thing. I have "The Big C." My heart pounded; my mouth went dry; and all the color went out of my world. All of a sudden, everything was moving in slow motion. My wife was with me when I retrieved my messages and she instantly knew what had happened from the expression on my face. "I have prostate cancer, honey," I said.

I told her I wasn't going to call the doctor and spoil the rest of our vacation. I just didn't want to hear those words from him, even though I knew what he was going to say. But my wife persuaded me otherwise. "Why torture yourself and me? You've got to make that call." I tried to come up with an argument to support my position, but I knew she was right.

So I made the call and here is what I heard: "Mr. Marckini, your biopsy results came back, and you have prostate cancer. Two of the eight samples tested positively for adenocarcinoma. The good news is that we caught it at an early stage. Less than five percent of your prostate is involved."

The rest of the conversation was a blur. After he told me I had cancer I didn't really hear anything else he said.

We set up an appointment for the following week so we could finish our vacation in Nantucket. But the vacation really ended with that phone call. We stayed a few more days, but my mind was on cancer, surgery, blood loss, impotence, incontinence . . . and death.

Communicating with Family and Friends

I remember telling two of our closest friends and fighting back tears as I gave them the details. This wasn't going to be easy. I was frightened, and it showed. My wife asked me if it would be easier for me if she told our other friends who were vacationing with us. Sheepishly, I said yes. It was awkward for a couple of days. But by the time vacation was over, we were discussing my prostate cancer with our friends, casually, over dinner.

Frequently, in the back of my mind, however, I could see the haunting image of my brother in the recovery room, and I pictured myself in his place. It was a nightmare.

Telling my two daughters I had prostate cancer was one of the most difficult things I've ever had to do. This was complicated by the fact that we were planning my younger daughter's wedding, only a few weeks away.

"Oh, my God," I thought, "Will I be able to walk her down the aisle?" It's amazing the things that go through your head when you get news like this.

I waited until vacation was over, when I could tell them face-to-face. I also wanted more time to get used to the idea, so I would sound matter-of-fact about it, and not worry them. After all, I kept telling myself, it *was* early stage cancer and I was only 57 years old and in excellent health.

My daughters handled the news well and committed their prayers and support, which was exactly what I needed. I received similar responses from my friends and relatives.

It was There All The Time

I later learned that cancer takes years to grow, and that it was certainly present in my prostate two years before, when I had my first biopsy. Then why didn't the doctor find it? Because he only took six samples, three in each lobe. Certainly if he had taken more samples, the chances of finding the cancer would have been much greater.

Some doctors, I discovered, routinely take eight samples, others take twelve, and some more progressive urologists remove twenty-four tissue samples. If you think about it, the chances of finding microscopic cancer cells increases manyfold with a larger number of samples.

Look at it this way: Picture a football stadium filled three feet deep with several billion white marbles – which represent normal, healthy cells. Now, from a plane, sprinkle a few hundred black marbles (representing cancer cells) over the stadium and mix them in with a bulldozer. Next picture yourself going into the stadium with a shovel blindfolded. What are your chances of finding some black marbles if you only remove six shovels-full of marbles? Pretty slim. Certainly the more samples, you take, the greater your chances of finding some of the black marbles. The same is true when doing a prostate biopsy.

Rising PSA tells you there *may* be cancer cells in your prostate. In early stage prostate cancer, there is typically no detectable tumor or lump on which to focus the biopsy needle. This is much different from other forms of cancer, such as breast cancer, where a lump or lesion is usually evident. With breast cancer, the biopsy needle can be directed to the suspicious area.

If there is cancer in your prostate, it is to your *great* advantage to find it early. Early cancer detection means a) more treatment options, b) better chance of a cure, and c) better quality of life after treatment.

A recent study published in the Daily University Science News pointed out that one in seven cancers are missed by biopsy sampling – all the more reason for increasing the number of samples taken.

If cancer is present, your PSA will continue to rise and you will be facing the unpleasant biopsy experience again. So, why put yourself through the "trauma" of multiple biopsies needlessly? If the cancer is there, you want to find it – and you want to find it early.

There is one more reason for taking a larger number of biopsy samples. If the pathology results do, in fact, come back negative, you are much more confident that there really is no cancer present, and you can rest easy.

Tip: If you are going to have a prostate biopsy, insist on a minimum of twelve samples. Twenty samples would be even better. And insist on local anesthesia to eliminate pain and discomfort.

Looking back, and knowing what I know now, here are some facts that would have altered my thinking and my approach to diagnosis:

1. My father had prostate cancer. This *doubled* my chance of being diagnosed.

2. My older brother was diagnosed with prostate cancer. With two close relatives having been diagnosed, my chances were *five times greater* than the average man.

3. The rapid rise in my PSA (more than 0.75 ng/ml in 1 year) was one more indicator that cancer was present more than two years before it was diagnosed.

4. When my brother was diagnosed, my PSA was in the high end of the normal range. Considering all the other factors, the probability I had prostate cancer was almost certain.

If I knew then what I know now, I would have insisted on a minimum 20-core biopsy, done under local anesthesia, and in all probability, my cancer would have been detected years earlier.

Why is this important? Simply because, the earlier you diagnose this disease, the higher the probability the cancer is still localized and curable. I was fortunate that mine was *still* discovered relatively early. However, if my doctor – or I – had been more alert, or better informed, I would have been diagnosed at a time that would have substantially improved my chance of a cure.

Tip: You must become your own advocate when it comes to protecting yourself from this disease. You must learn what you need to know about what puts you at higher risk for prostate cancer. You must take responsibility for tracking your own PSA. You must have a competent physician working with you in this process. The information presented in this book will teach you how to do all of these things.

CHAPTER 4

My Preliminary Research

Out of your vulnerabilities will come your strength.
-- Sigmund Freud

As an engineer, I was accustomed to collecting data, dealing with technical information, evaluating pros and cons of options, and making decisions. My problem, however, was not a lack of information; it was the opposite – an overwhelming *abundance* of information. And most disconcerting, in my early research, was the fact that no option seemed to emerge as the preferred choice. They all had significant drawbacks.

Between the time I received the phone call with the diagnosis, and my first meeting with the urologist, I devoured everything I could find on prostate cancer treatment. I wanted to be prepared for the meeting with all the information I could gather, including a list of all the important questions.

I began by making calls to all the people I knew who had dealt with this dreaded disease. Each one of them gave me the name of two or three people they knew who were treated for prostate cancer. The list grew and grew, and there was one common theme. All these men had chosen surgery – radical prostatectomy. Was it going to be as simple as this?

But what about the promise I made myself that day in the recovery room, standing beside my brother following his surgery?

Tip: When doing your own research, make sure you talk with several men who have been treated by each of the major treatment options, not just surgery. I cannot overemphasize how important this is in your own personal treatment decision. Spend time with them. Take them out to lunch if possible. Much information comes out after the first few minutes of polite conversation.

With the exception of one of these men, they all informed me of the seriousness of the surgery, the discomfort they experienced following their treatment, and the lingering side effects they were dealing with. The most common side effect reported was partial to complete loss of sexual potency, followed closely by varying degrees of incontinence, or loss of bladder control. One individual, a healthy, athletic 63 year-old told me the operation was "no big deal," that he experienced no side effects, and that he felt he had made the right decision. My research continued.

While I made my telephone calls, I continued to work the Internet. I discovered that surgery was the most common treatment recommended by urologists, followed by various forms of radiation including external beam (x-ray) radiation and brachytherapy (radioactive seed implantation). There was also reference to cryoablation using liquid nitrogen to kill the cancer by freezing it.

Another approach chosen by some men is essentially doing nothing, except monitoring the situation. This is called "Watchful Waiting," or "Active Surveillance." Under certain circumstances this can be the best approach.

Somewhere in the thousands of pages of Internet literature there was a passing reference to a treatment called proton beam therapy. The information was limited in scope and offered minimal details. At the time I assumed this to be an experimental treatment and, therefore, placed the information I downloaded on proton therapy off to the side in my office.

My search continued.

Help from the Caribbean

Early in this process I received a call from a good friend, who was retired and living on his sailboat in the Caribbean. Larry had been diagnosed with prostate cancer a year before, and had chosen surgery on his urologist's recommendation. He also suffered some of the typical side effects. I had e-mailed Larry notifying him of my diagnosis. He received my message on his wireless computer system somewhere off the coast of Grenada. A couple of days later he called me.

Larry reinforced my resolve to try to find an alternative to surgery as he related to me details of his lingering side effects. In the same conversation he told me the story of his friend Max, a Caribbean boating acquaintance who had recently been treated for prostate cancer. I didn't realize it at the time, but this conversation turned out to be a major turning point in my search for the best treatment.

Proton Treatment is Real

Larry told me that he and Max had been treated for prostate cancer at about the same time. Weeks later, when both were back in the Caribbean, Larry was out for his daily walk, still tender from his surgery, when Max jogged by. Larry was dumbfounded, as he had assumed Max had also chosen surgery.

When Larry inquired, he learned that Max had chosen proton therapy, and this treatment involved no pain, no blood loss, no trauma and no discomfort. Max, in fact, told Larry he jogged each day while he was in treatment.

When Larry heard this, he couldn't wait to tell me about his discovery. He knew I was doing research, and needed to make a treatment decision. He also knew I was searching for an alternative to surgery.

I told Larry I had heard about proton treatment, but I hadn't really gotten into it in much detail. He told me that although this procedure was relatively new, he heard it was not experimental, the cure rates were comparable to surgery, and it was covered by medical insurance. Most exciting to me was the fact that Max reported experiencing no side effects whatsoever.

During the phone conversation with Larry, I dug through my research material and found the scant, few pages I had downloaded from the Internet on proton treatment. The information was interesting, but after reading it I still had more questions than answers.

I asked Larry for Max's cell phone number and called him. We spent about 45 minutes on the phone and he answered all my questions. Max was a well-educated, successful, retired businessman, and as such, his decision to choose proton gave this option much credence. He had done his homework. His urologist had recommended surgery, but Max put that on hold until he evaluated all the options. He read everything he could on the subject, and he visited Loma Linda University Medical Center (LLUMC) in Southern California to meet with the doctors and staff.

Max recounted the details of his treatment and told me about his life changing experience in Southern California.

When I finished talking with Max I was excited. "Maybe this is it," I thought. But being a "recovering engineer," I knew I had a lot more work to do.

In the meantime I had to meet with my urologist for the first time since my positive biopsy. I knew from my brother's experience that the doctor would recommend surgery. I wanted to ask the right questions, so I did a quick study of this procedure, called radical prostatectomy.

Meeting with My Urologist

The day came, and my wife and I met with my urologist – one of the finest in his profession in the country. He pointed out that I was fortunate, that my cancer was early stage. He told me that my tumor stage was T1c and my Gleason score was "only a 3+2, or 5." The way he said this, sounded like I should feel good about it. I was just beginning to learn about Gleason score and realized this was in the middle of the range, but I didn't know much more than that.

Next he told me that my physical health and relative youth (57 years old!) made me an ideal candidate for surgery, with an excellent chance of full recovery. He even used a term I would hear several more times during my due diligence. He told me I was the "poster boy" for radical prostatectomy (RP).

When I asked about alternatives to surgery, he indicated there were a few, but I should only seriously consider two, brachytherapy (seeds) or external beam radiation therapy (EBRT). He gave me the name of physicians in these specialties and suggested I speak with them.

"If I choose surgery doctor, when could you do it?" I asked. "No sooner than four weeks from now, as you need to bank four units of your own blood," he replied. Again, I pictured my brother in the recovery room after losing six pints of blood.

I thought it was time to ask him the question that was burning in my mind. "Doctor, I've been doing some research and I came across something called 'proton therapy,' and it looks quite interesting."

His reaction caught me totally off guard. He brushed it off and said, "That's experimental. You could damage your rectum and wind up needing a colostomy."

I was devastated. A colostomy, I knew was a surgical procedure, where a section of the colon is brought out through an opening in the abdomen. Stools pass into a small bag fastened over the opening.

I felt like I had been kicked in the stomach. That statement certainly deflated my enthusiasm for the treatment that seemed so right for me. But I pressed on, asking more questions about proton. I told him about what I had read, and what I had heard from a former patient. He changed the subject and told us to go home and think about the three "legitimate" options we had discussed. We left with some documents to read and forms to sign.

Driving home, I began to think that what I had been reading about proton therapy was all hype. Maybe I was being unrealistic to think I could get through this thing without the trauma and side effects of the more "conventional" treatments. "After all," I thought, I have one of the best urologists in the northeast, and he would be the 'expert' in these matters."

I later discovered that other patients received similar responses from their urologists when asked about proton therapy. I also learned the sad fact that most general practitioners and urologists are unfamiliar with proton technology. This is changing.

After replaying in my mind, the events of the meeting with my urologist, it started to become clear to me. He really couldn't answer my questions about proton therapy, because he really didn't know much about it. Yet, a hospital in Southern California spent $100 Million on this technology in the late 1980s, and has treated thousands of patients over the past several years, with excellent results. And, at least two other major medical centers, including Massachusetts General Hospital – right in my doctor's back yard – were building Proton treatment centers. This treatment *had* to be legitimate.

This was a major realization for me, and it reaffirmed my earlier conclusion that *I needed to take charge of the treatment decision*. I could not leave this critical decision in the hands of my urologist – and no man should. I had lived my whole life believing that, "The doctor always knows best." And I learned during this journey, this is not always true. Our doctors might, in good faith, feel they are making the best recommendation, but that is not always the case, especially when it comes to treating prostate cancer.

Tip: If you get nothing more from this book than this, it will have been worth your investment: Take charge of your treatment decision. Do not rely on your urologist alone. He or she is fundamentally a surgeon. That's what they know best and that is typically what they recommend. It may not be best for you. There are alternatives and each of them should be evaluated before you make your treatment decision.

I had left my urologist's office even more confused and anxious than when I entered. But I found myself more determined than ever to continue my search for the *right* treatment for me.

The packet of information my urologist gave me included information about the surgical procedure, called radical prostatectomy, as well as some statistics on the "gold standard," as it is often called.

Among these papers was a consent form that described possible complications and side effects from surgery. These included the following:

- Impotence (inability to maintain an erection)

- Incontinence (inability to maintain urinary control)

- Strictures of bladder and/or urethra requiring stretching or further procedures

- Damage to rectal wall (requiring temporary colostomy)

- No guarantee of cancer cure

- Infection of incision requiring further treatment

- Emboli (blood clots) from veins into the lung (rare, serious)

At this point, I remember saying to my wife, "I think I'll continue my research."

CHAPTER 5

Understanding My Diagnosis

"Your life today is the result of your attitude and the decisions you made yesterday. Your life tomorrow will be the result of your attitude and decisions you make today." -- Unknown

Cancer Grading and Staging

The next thing I needed to know was what the doctor meant by cancer stage and grade. And why should I feel good about having a T1c, Gleason 5 diagnosis?

Here is what I learned about the difference between stage and grade:

Grade describes how closely the individual cancer cells resemble normal cells of the same type, thus giving an indication of how fast the cancer is growing.

Stage describes the extent of the cancer in your body, or how far the cancer has spread.

Grading – Gleason Score

So, why should I feel good about a 3 + 2 = 5? I learned that biopsy samples are examined under a microscope by a pathologist. The shape and form of the cells are a clear indication of a pattern that indicates the level of aggressiveness of the cancer. Figure 5-1 shows what the pathologist sees under a microscope when he/she is looking at the five patterns, or levels, of prostate cancer.

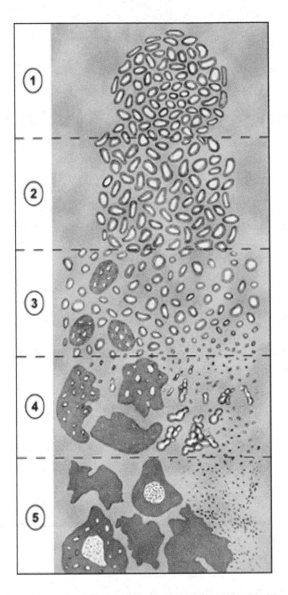

Source: American Journal of Surgical Pathology, Volume 29, Number 9, September 2005. *The 2005 International Society of Urological Pathology (ISUP) Consensus Conference on Gleason Grading of Prostatic Carcinoma*, Jonathan Epstein, MD, William C. Allsbrook, Jr, MD, Mahul B. Admin, AD, and Lars Edgevad, MD, PhD, and the ISUP Grading Committee

Pattern 1. Well-differentiated cells that look similar to normal cells. These cells are typically round, closely packed and have well-defined edges.

Pattern 2. Still well-differentiated, but slightly less so than Pattern 1 cells. Also more loosely packed and may have less well-defined edges.

Pattern 3. Moderately differentiated. These may be medium sized cells, irregularly shaped, not forming chains or cords.

Pattern 4. These are glands or cells of all sizes fused into cords or chains.

Pattern 5. Similar to 4, but with large clear cancer cells.

The pathologist examines all the biopsy samples and scores each. He then takes the two most prominent Gleason patterns and adds them together – in my case 3 + 2, for a Gleason score of 5. The maximum Gleason score is 10 (5 + 5) and is indicative of a most aggressive cancer. Overall, Gleason scores in the 2 to 4 range are considered very early stage. Scores in the 8 to 10 range implies later stage. My score of 5 put me on the high end of early stage.

A Gleason score of 3 + 2 = 5 has a dominant, moderately differentiated pattern (i.e., pattern 3) and a less dominant, well-differentiated pattern (i.e., pattern 2). A 4+3=7 Gleason score means that a poorly differentiated component (pattern 4) is dominant. If 95% or more of the tumor has the same characteristic pattern, then the same number is counted twice. A moderately differentiated tumor, for example, would therefore be a 3+3=6 Gleason score.

A Gleason score of 2 + 2 or 2 + 1, indicates that the tumor is well differentiated – looks much like a normal cell of the same type – is able to carry out some of the functions of a normal cell and has a low probability of spreading or metastasis in the near future. A score of 3 + 2 or 3 + 4, indicates a moderate probability of metastasis, and a Gleason score of 4 + 4 or 5 + 5, indicates a more aggressive cancer with higher probability of metastasis.

Staging

I learned in my research that there are two commonly used staging systems – ABCD and TNM. The ABCD system has been used the longest, but is slowly being replaced by the TNM staging system, which seems to be more commonly used today. TNM staging is usually combined with a number such as 1, 2, or 3. The three letters T, N and M, respectively describe the prostate *T*umor, the lymph *N*odes and *M*etastasis or distant spread of the disease.

ABCD Staging

Stage A cancers have no symptoms, and there is no detectable abnormality by DRE. Cancer is confined to the prostate and is accidentally discovered while surgery is being performed for other reasons.

Stage B cancers are usually discovered by needle biopsy that is done as a result of rising PSA or tumor felt by DRE.

Stage C cancer cells have spread outside the prostate capsule to the surrounding tissue and possibly the seminal vesicles, which are the glands that produce the semen.

Stage D cancer cells have spread or metastasized to lymph nodes, organs or tissue distant from the prostate. This could include the liver, bones or lungs.

TNM Staging

T1a is similar to Stage A, in that there are no symptoms and it is accidentally discovered. These cancers are low grade and involve less than 5% of the tissue sampled

T1b is also similar to Stage A, but the cancer cells can be either low or high grade and involve more than 5% of the tissue sampled.

44

T1c was my cancer stage. This cancer is similar to Stage B. The tumor is detected by needle biopsy as a result of elevated PSA.

T2a cancer involves only one lobe of the prostate and can be felt by DRE.

T2b cancer involves more that half of one lobe, but not both sides of the prostate.

T2c involves both lobes

T3a is similar to Stage C and indicates that the cancer has spread beyond the capsule on one side of the gland.

T3b cancer has spread beyond the prostate capsule on both sides.

T4a indicates that the cancer has spread into adjacent structures such as the bladder, sphincter or rectum.

NX Regional lymph nodes cannot be assessed

NO No regional lymph node metastasis

N1 is similar to Stage D. Cancer cells have extended to a single pelvic lymph node 2 cm or less in size.

N2 cells are in a single pelvic lymph node greater than 2 cm in size

N3 cells have spread to any pelvic lymph node with more than 5 cm in greatest dimension.

M1 indicates distant metastasis to other parts of the body outside of the pelvic region.

Understanding this whole table is a little daunting at first. I settled on just understanding my own staging level, which was T1c, with no "N" and no "M," thank God. Again, my T1c indicated the cancer was discovered by needle biopsy that was performed as a result of rising PSA, and there was no "palpable" tumor – i.e. no tumor felt by digital rectal exam. The vast majority of diagnosed prostate cancers, I later discovered, fall into the T1/T2 category.

Second Pathology Report

Somewhere in my research I learned that a pathologists reading of biopsy slides under a microscope is a subjective process, and it's a good idea to have your slides read by a second pathology lab. So I called my urologist and made the request. He agreed that it was a wise move and sent my slides to another pathology lab in Boston.

A week later I was sorry I had made the request. The second lab read my slides as a 3 + 3, or Gleason score 6. This meant they felt my two most prominent patterns of cancer were at level 3. Now what? Which lab was right? Was I a Gleason 5 or 6? In my case, it didn't matter a whole lot.

This experience taught me, however, the importance of getting a second opinion from another pathologist on your biopsy slides. Why? Because some differences might dictate different approaches to treating the cancer, or perhaps even cause you to rule out a particular treatment method. A Gleason 8 versus a Gleason 7, for example, could indicate a much higher probability of the cancer spreading beyond the gland. In this case, a patient may want to favor an approach that treats the entire prostate bed rather than the prostate alone.

Tip: Since the reading of biopsy slides is a subjective process, have your slides read by at least two different laboratories. The Appendix includes a listing of the premier pathology labs in the U.S.

X-rays, Rads and Gray

Our next planned stop was with a Radiation Oncologist. But before that meeting, I had some more studying to do. I needed the answers to some questions: How does radiation kill cancer? What kind of radiation is used? How much radiation is necessary? Do they still use the term "Rads" to measure radiation as they did when I was in college? How do they prevent damage to healthy organs and tissues when bombarding my private parts with this deadly beam?

I didn't answer all those questions before the next appointment, but I expanded my knowledge in a couple of areas. I learned that X-ray radiation is also called "photon radiation," and that X-rays are a form of electromagnetic radiation, similar to radio waves and visible light, but with much shorter wavelength. X-rays, or photons, have no mass, and they travel at the speed of light. They interact electrically with atoms that make up the cells in our bodies, even though they have no net electrical charge.

The International System of Measurement (SI) has chosen the term Cobalt Gray, or more commonly, Gray (abbreviated "Gy") as the radiation unit of measurement. More correctly, the Gy is the unit of *absorbed* dose. One Gy is equivalent to 100 Rads, the term I was more familiar with from college physics.

Meeting with a Radiation Oncologist

Armed with this new information, my wife and I met with another Boston physician who specialized in conformal external beam radiation therapy (EBRT). Here I learned I was an "ideal candidate for EBRT," a "poster boy," in fact. This was beginning to get interesting. How could I be the "poster boy" for both surgery and EBRT?

I began asking questions. How much radiation would I be receiving? What are my chances of survival? What is the probability of impotence, incontinence, rectal damage, and other side effects?

I learned that at that time, late 2000, they typically delivered about 75 Gy of photon (X-ray) radiation to the tumor site. I also learned that, in order to minimize collateral radiation damage to other parts of my body, they would be sending in the radiation beam from several different angles around the perimeter of my pelvic region. I did a quick mental inventory of important body parts in my pelvic region, and I remember feeling nauseous.

"What about side effects?" I asked. "Short term, you might experience some urinary urgency, urinary burning and fatigue. The most common long-term side effects are impotence, incontinence and rectal damage. There could also be urethra strictures."

Noticing the beads of perspiration, loss of color, and panicked look on my face, the doctor smiled and told me that, because of my age and physical condition, I was unlikely to experience all these things. I would probably come through this with only mild forms of these side effects. I remember thinking, "How can I be mildly incontinent? Maybe I'd only need two diapers a day instead of five?"

It was during this meeting that I realized I feared incontinence the most. True, I was only 57, and my wife and I still enjoyed regular sexual activity. Certainly, the loss of sexual potency would be terrible. But loss of bladder control, "That's what happens to old people," I thought, "in nursing homes!" I had 25 to 30 more years to live. I didn't want to spend that time in diapers. Could he guarantee I wouldn't be incontinent? "Sorry, but I can't," he said.

Brachytherapist Meeting

Gaining in knowledge (and new levels of fear), my wife and I next met with a prominent Boston oncologist who specialized in brachytherapy, or radioactive seed implants.

This physician told me I was an ideal candidate for seeds. And, in fact, considering my cancer stage, age, prostate size, and physical health, he said, "You are a perfect candidate for seeds." I remember commenting, "Would you say I'm the 'poster boy' for seeds?" He responded, "You could say that." Terrific, now I'm the poster boy for surgery, EBRT, and seeds. What more could I ask for?

He then described the procedure in great detail and told me my chances for a cure were very good. The side effects, he explained were similar to those of EBRT, but with much less radiation exposure to my torso, since all the radiation would be coming from inside my prostate. He also told me about the possibility of seed migration, and that, since I would be radioactive for a few months, I'd have to be careful about being near young children and pregnant women.

I took the opportunity of asking this doctor about Proton Therapy. He had some familiarity with this modality, but not a lot. He noted that protons are a type of radiation, and that radiation does, in fact kill cancer, so, "It's probably a viable treatment option."

Before our meeting ended, I decided to confront this 'poster boy' issue head on. "I have a question," I said, "I set you up earlier on this 'poster boy' issue. You're the third doctor who's told me I was the 'poster boy' for his treatment. How can I possibly be the 'poster boy' for surgery, EBRT and brachytherapy?" His answer was a revelation. He smiled and said, "Considering your age, cancer stage and physical health, whatever you choose for treatment, whether it be surgery, seeds, EBRT, cryotherapy, or proton radiation, it will most likely work for you – all with about the same, excellent chances of a cure. So learn what you can about each option, especially side effects and quality of life issues, and choose the one that best meets your needs."

I felt a thousand pound weight lifted from my shoulders. This took the pressure off surgery and gave me the incentive to keep all options on the table, and to crank up my research. My optimism was back.

CHAPTER 6

Investigating Treatment Options

"When thinking won't cure fear, action will."
-- William Clement Stone

Now My Research Gets Serious

Where should I go to fill in the gaps, to find out more about the specifics of each option, and especially the dreaded side effects? Should I focus on books, the Internet, or word of mouth? I learned that all three would serve as important information sources, but none more valuable than my personal interviews of former patients.

Books and magazine articles are generally thoroughly researched, well organized, refined documentations about medical research and individual case histories. The quality of information is generally good, as publishers demand that quality work is distributed under their names. I read several books and journals on prostate cancer prevention, detection, and treatment.

I found the Internet rich with information on prostate cancer. Topics tend to be specific and the technology presented is usually current. For example, you can gather considerable information on something as specific as Free PSA or the impact of diet and nutrition on prostate cancer prevention. There are also websites available where people can go to chat with others who are recently diagnosed patients, treated patients, or doctors involved in diagnosing and treating prostate cancer. A list of these websites is presented in the appendix.

I spent days reading everything I could find about Radical Prostatectomy, all forms of external beam radiation therapy, brachytherapy (seed implant), cryosurgery or cryoablation; as well as hormone treatment and watchful waiting.

Talk with the Customer

I have always been a believer in evaluating a product or service by checking with the customer. Gaining access to former patients in some cases was a challenge, but my persistence and determination prevailed. Some of my best information came from interviewing men who had chosen different options.

Information I gathered in my research fills several boxes and a substantial portion of my computer hard drive. I will not attempt to regurgitate everything I learned in my research. Instead, I will summarize in simple terms, the fundamentals, along with my assessment of the pros and cons of each option.

1. SURGERY (Radical Prostatectomy)

I frequently heard surgery referred to as the "Gold Standard" of prostate cancer treatments. It has been the most common treatment option prescribed by doctors and chosen by patients over the years. The theory is that if the cancer is confined to the prostate and this gland is surgically removed, there is no chance for the cancer to spread to other parts of the body. This is true, but there is a major qualifier here. It is the words "if the cancer is confined to the prostate." I would later find that there is reasonable probability, even for early stage cancer patients like myself that microscopic cancer cells have escaped the prostate gland. And when this happens, it usually "hangs around" the prostate capsule surface for some time before it eventually migrates to the lymph nodes and then gets transmitted to other parts of the body (metastasis).

Radical prostatectomy is *major* surgery. It is one of the most challenging operations in urology. Surgery is not suited for elderly men or men who are in poor or marginal physical condition. Men with certain heart problems for example, might not want to subject themselves to the trauma of surgery.

Surgery can carry undesirable side effects including impotence and incontinence. Additionally, since the cancer is not always confined to the prostate, a certain percentage of patients who undergo this procedure require re-treatment when the cancer returns. The re-treatment usually involves one of the other three options.

I had first hand knowledge of this option, having observed my brother's case. Also, several friends and acquaintances had chosen surgery. I made it a point to speak with all of them.

From my research I learned that the procedure involved preparation, which usually included banking a few pints of the patient's own blood over a one-month period. This was for the inevitable blood loss that accompanies this major surgery. The patient is typically placed under general anesthesia. An intravenous tube is inserted in the arm to provide fluids until the patient is able to eat and drink. Oxygen is administered until blood oxygen level is normalized. And a small drain is placed in the incision to remove fluid following surgery.

The prostate is located deep within the pelvis and is surrounded by organs and structures that are vulnerable to injury. This includes the bladder, the rectum and nerve bundles that are essential for male potency. An incision is made between the penis and navel. Next a major vein system is carefully severed and the urethra is cut making sure not to damage the urethral sphincter that controls urination.

The doctor then makes the decision as to how much, if any, of the nerve bundles that surround the prostate can be spared. It is these nerve bundles that control erectile function. The surgeon next separates the prostate from the bladder and removes the seminal vesicles and surrounding tissue. Finally the doctor reattaches the bladder and urethra and begins the process of suturing up the patient.

During the procedure a catheter is inserted into the penis in order to drain urine from the bladder. The catheter remains in place for two to three weeks.

Recuperation from surgery generally takes from one to three months. During that time the patient must deal with bowel issues, catheter management and removal, and temporary incontinence.

Cure rates with all forms of treatment vary by cancer stage and many other factors. Certainly younger, healthier men with early stage prostate cancer will see higher cure rates than average.

Most of the men I interviewed told me they had no regrets for having chosen surgery, although several said things like, "I hope I'll never have to go through something like that again." A few were incontinent, or marginally continent, and most seemed reluctant to talk about impotence. Sexual potency is something we males equate to our "manhood," and thus, when it diminishes we aren't always honest about our status. Those who did admit to impotence seemed to be split into two groups. One group was completely impotent with erectile dysfunction and no libido. The other group used medications (e.g. Viagra), devices (pumps), injections, or implants with varying degrees of success.

Because men are so reluctant to talk about loss of sexual potency, I suspect the impotency numbers reported for *all* treatment options are understated.

While most of the surgery patients I interviewed seemed to be doing well, three had experienced relapses, and had undergone follow-up salvage treatments, radiation and/or hormone therapy. One had a urethral stricture resulting from his surgery and had to undergo a "Roto-Rooter procedure" as he described it. One experienced an infection that caused much discomfort for weeks following surgery. Another told me of an acquaintance who had surgery and had serious complications from blood clots.

I really didn't want to have surgery, and my interviews helped with my decision.

Here is What I Learned are the Advantages of Surgery:

- Surgery is called the "Gold Standard" because it is the oldest and most common treatment for prostate cancer. There is more statistical data available on cure rates and side effects for surgery than any other treatment option.

- For some men, there is a psychological benefit knowing the cancerous gland has been removed from their body.

- *If* the cancer is confined to the prostate, it is gone for good.

And the Disadvantages of Surgery:

- Surgery requires hospitalization and anesthesia. A radical prostatectomy is *major* surgery, which means trauma and probable blood loss.

- There is always a risk of infection, and even death from major surgery. I read that one-half of 1% of men treated with surgery die on the operating table – that's one out of every 200.

- There is a long recuperation period following surgery – usually two or three months before full physical activity can be resumed. Fatigue sometimes lasts for a year or more.

- Surgery carries a 60% to 90% chance of impotence. Most literature reports a 75% chance of impotency, or three out of four men. Nerve sparing surgeons report impotence statistics in the 10% to 25% range, but many doubt the validity of these claims. Age, general health, and the experience of the surgeon are all important factors here.

- Incontinence occurs in 20% to 40% of the cases. Patient age and the physician's skills are also factors.

- Other less common side effects are strictures of the bladder or urethra, damage to the rectal wall, and blood clots.

- Surgery has little value if the cancer has progressed beyond the prostate. This usually cannot be seen at the time of surgery. If found later it requires follow-up salvage treatment.

- Surgery is heavily practitioner dependent. Many urologists claim to do "nerve sparing surgery." But different doctors, with different levels of experience, using different techniques have a broad range of outcomes. Despite what some physician's say, a radical prostatectomy is not "routine surgery."

Tip: Thousands of urologists do radical prostatectomies every day. The operation is serious and delicate. Not all doctors employ the same techniques. Many doctors claim to do "nerve sparing surgery," implying that they make every attempt to save the nerve bundles necessary for sexual function. Be sure to check out the doctor who will do your surgery. How many procedures has he or she done? Speak to ten or fifteen men who have been operated on by this surgeon. What have been their results and side effects? Choose only the most experienced and successful doctor for this critically important procedure.

An alternative to "open prostate surgery" as described above is Laparoscopic Radical Prostatectomy (LRP). This is relatively new and is a substantially more difficult procedure. Louis Kavoussi, a pioneering laparoscopic surgeon, who is Vice Chairman of Urology at Johns Hopkins Medical Center did twenty of these procedures and stopped, because he didn't think the operation, which took an average of nine hours, was superior to open surgery.

While LRP, which is gaining in popularity, generally involves less blood loss and results in shorter recovery times, the complications can be more severe. Rectal injury, for example, is more common with the laparoscopic procedure, according to an article in the June 16, 2003 issue of NEWSWEEK Magazine.

DaVinci Robotic Laparoscopic Radical Prostatectomy is also gaining in popularity. However, based on recently published information and discussions with former patients, there is no reason to believe that complications and side effects will be appreciably different from conventional LRP.

The Center for the Advancement of Health concluded in an August 2005 study that, "Prostate cancer patients' biggest concerns -- after cure -- are the possible side effects of surgery, including urinary incontinence and sexual impotency. Data on these side effects from robotically assisted prostatectomy were sketchy at best, and no evidence was available to indicate that any surgical method emerged as better than another for these side effects."

The results of this study were posted on the National Prostate Cancer Coalition website.

2. EXTERNAL BEAM RADIATION

Through my research and conversations with radiation oncologists I learned several interesting things about radiation and cancer:

1. Radiation has been used to kill cancer for more than 60 years.
2. Urologists are reluctant to operate on men older than 65 to 70 – and radiation is usually the treatment of choice in these cases.
3. Radiation is often prescribed for men with health issues that might be compromised or exacerbated by the trauma of surgery.
4. Radiation is commonly used as a salvage treatment when surgery fails.
5. Radiation is a standard treatment for "localized" (non-metastasized) prostate cancer. This typically includes stages T1 through T3, or A, B and C.
6. The higher the radiation dose, the better the chance of a cure.

All forms of radiation kill cancer the same way. They cause damage to the cancer cell's DNA structure. The cells live out their "normal" life span, but the radiation damage prevents them from growing and dividing, and they eventually die off. This phenomenon is referred to as programmed cell death, or "apoptosis."

There are different forms of radiation, both in physical characteristics and in method of delivery to the cancer. I learned it is important to understand these differences as the impact on quality of life following treatment can vary depending on the option chosen.

The four types of radiation used to kill cancer are X-rays (or photons), protons, gamma rays, and neutrons. Gamma rays and neutrons are seldom used, so I am limiting my discussions to X-rays/photons and protons.

It is important to understand the fundamental difference between these two types of radiation. In simplest terms, photon (X-ray) radiation is at its maximum intensity where it *enters* the body. It loses energy on the way to the tumor site, thus radiating everything in its path as it travels into the body, passing through the tumor site and then out of the body. For this reason, multiple body entry points must be selected to reduce collateral damage to healthy tissue and organs.

Proton radiation loses a small portion of its energy on the way to the tumor site, deposits the bulk of its energy on the target volume, and has a zero exit dose. This results in less radiation damage to healthy tissues and organs.

Radiation treatment is painless, tasteless, and has no smell. Radiation treatment goals can be either palliative (to improve the quality of life in a patient with terminal or irreversible cancer) or curative (to attempt to cure or rid a patient of their cancer). My research focused on the latter.

Conventional External Beam Radiation

Conventional external beam radiation therapy (EBRT) involves directing high-energy photons (x-rays) to the cancer site.

Instead of administering all the radiation in one dose, which would cause serious, irreparable harm, it is delivered in small "fractions" over an extended period of time. Each treatment lasts only a few minutes and is painless. The entry point of the radiation is usually varied in order to minimize damage to healthy tissue. The challenge with all forms of radiation is delivering maximum dosage to the cancer site without damaging surrounding healthy tissue and organs.

Common to all forms of external beam radiation is the planning process. It is important to precisely pinpoint the treatment target volume and plan the treatment series. In treating prostate cancer, physicians typically prescribe about 40 treatments. Treatment sessions usually last about 15 to 20 minutes, once a day, five days a week.

Three Dimensional Conformal Radiation Therapy (3D-CRT)

As the name implies, this method of delivering photons involves the use of computers to accurately map the prostate area. The patient is immobilized and radiation is delivered from multiple angles. The radiation beam is shaped to include a 3-dimensional anatomic configuration of the prostate. The intent with Conformal

Radiation Therapy is to target the tumor volume more precisely and to minimize damage to surrounding organs and tissue. 3D-CRT allows higher doses of radiation to the prostate, with less normal tissue complications than conventional EBRT.

Intensity Modulated Radiation Therapy (IMRT)

IMRT is also a relatively new technology and is growing in popularity. Other forms of photon radiation use a single radiation beam of fixed energy level. IMRT varies the energy level over the field being treated by using multiple beams of varying intensity. The higher intensity beams are directed at the thicker part of the tumor volume, and the lower intensity beams are aimed at thinner segments. Specialized equipment costing about $1 million is required to administer this treatment. Because it is more precisely focused, IMRT reduces the amount of radiation exposure to surrounding healthy tissue, and reportedly produces fewer side effects than EBRT or 3D-CRT.

Advantages of Radiation Therapy:

- Data suggests the long term cure rates for all forms of external radiation are equivalent to surgery.
- External radiation therapy is non-invasive. There is no pain, trauma or blood loss during treatment.
- Hospitalization is not required. Treatment is done on an out-patient basis.

Disadvantages of Radiation Therapy:

- Eight to nine weeks of treatment are necessary to safely deliver all the radiation necessary to kill the cancer.
- The literature reports 30% to 60% of the patients who choose external beam radiation therapy experience some degree of impotence after completing treatment. Although this figure is high, it is generally lower than the surgical alternative. Age,

general health and the specific radiation treatment chosen all impact this statistic.

- Incontinence has been reported in 5% to 20% of cases, again depending on many factors.
- Other less common side effects include rectal damage and urethra constrictions from scar tissue.

Tip: The term incontinence is often used to describe anything ranging from minimal leakage to complete loss of bladder control. When you are talking with a doctor or interviewing a former patient, be sure you understand what they mean by the term incontinence. For example, some men I interviewed reported no incontinence, but later admitted having to wear pads while sleeping or leaking during any significant physical exertion. Others experience "stress incontinence," or loss of urine during physical activity, such as coughing, sneezing, laughing or exercise.

Short-term side effects from external beam radiation may include fatigue, skin irritation, frequent and painful urination, diarrhea, upset stomach, and rectal bleeding.

3. BRACHYTHERAPY (Radioactive Seeds)

This technique involves delivering radiation to the tumor site from *within* the prostate. I learned that if I chose this option, a physician would surgically implant 50 to 125 tiny radioactive seeds directly into my prostate gland. These seeds emit low levels of radiation from a few weeks to several months, depending on the type of seeds used.

The patient is given a spinal or general anesthesia, and hollow needles containing the seeds are inserted into the prostate through the perineum, the area between the scrotum and the anus. Different imaging techniques are used by doctors to place the rice-sized seeds in the proper position within the gland.

The procedure takes two to three hours to perform. A catheter is inserted through the penis to drain the bladder, and the patient typically spends one night in the hospital. The next day, the catheter is removed and the patient goes home. Pain and discomfort are nominal, and the patient usually resumes normal activities in a few days. Follow-up visits to the hospital are required for several weeks.

Because of the short treatment time, minimal trauma and rapid recovery, brachytherapy is gaining in popularity, particularly among younger men whose busy work schedules would be disrupted by the alternative treatment options.

Advantages of Brachytherapy:

- Cure rates comparable to surgery and external beam radiation options.
- Short hospitalization stay and quick recuperation period.
- Although a surgical procedure, brachytherapy is significantly less invasive than surgery. Trauma is minimal and there is essentially no blood loss.
- Since the radiation source is within the prostate gland, there is generally less radiation damage to other organs and tissue.

Disadvantages of Brachytherapy:

- Risks associated with spinal or general anesthesia.
- The risk of impotence and incontinence is comparable to external radiation.
- Since the seeds remain in place indefinitely, they continue to emit low levels of radiation for several weeks to months. For this reason, patients are advised not to have close contact with pregnant women or young children for a few months.
- It is common for seeds to dislodge and migrate to other parts of the body including the lungs. The long-term impact of this is not known.
- Uncertainty as to whether sufficient dosage will reach the periphery of the gland where tumor recurrence/spread tends to occur.
- Initial training in this procedure was somewhat limited and standardization was lacking.
- Seeds can be passed in the semen to a partner during intercourse.

- One nuclear radiation expert has reported that during the first few weeks following seed implant, the patient may trigger highly sensitive terrorist alarms at airports.

There is conflicting information on brachytherapy side effects. Most of the literature seems to indicate that side effects are comparable to external beam radiation therapy. However, according to a study conducted by Dr. Jeff Michalski, Assistant Professor of Radiation Oncology at the Washington University School of Medicine, "Patients who underwent brachytherapy reported significantly more urinary, sexual and bowel problems than men treated with external-beam radiation."

An article in the August 2001 Journal of Urology cited incontinence levels of up to 45% following brachytherapy.

On the subject of seed migration, the Journal of Urology (Urology 2002;59:555-559) reported that with brachytherapy, in approximately 36% of the cases, a small number of radioactive seeds became dislodged and migrated to the lungs. Other studies have reported brachytherapy seeds migrating to the coronary artery. And, while there is no evidence of short-term harm, the long-term effects are not yet known. Some work has been done to string seeds together to prevent migration, but little is known of the success of the technique at this writing.

The urethra, which channels urine and semen outside the body, runs through the center of the prostate gland. The center of the gland receives a much higher dose of radiation with brachytherapy, than with any other form of radiation therapy. This may be the reason for higher levels of urinary problems reported with brachytherapy.

The most important thing I learned about brachytherapy is that it is extremely practitioner dependent. A small number of physicians who use advanced imaging techniques, and do a large number of procedures, have significantly better results than the others.

Tip: A growing number of doctors are now performing this relatively new procedure. Precise placement of the radioactive seeds is the key to success. Different visualization and placement techniques are used by different doctors. If you choose this procedure, select one of the few doctors who utilize the most up-to-date technology and have done hundreds of procedures. Do your homework!

Brachytherapy cannot be performed on men with significantly enlarged prostates, and is usually limited to stage A and B cancers.

The premier brachytherapy practitioners in the world are reported to be Dr. John Blasko and Dr. Peter Grimm at the Seattle Prostate Cancer Institute.

Andy Grove and Brachytherapy

Andy Grove was president and CEO of Intel, a man of considerable intellect and financial means. Somewhere on the Internet I saw a reference to an article in Fortune Magazine about his journey with prostate cancer. He had chosen hormones plus High Dose Rate Brachytherapy and EBRT, commonly referred to as HDR and wrote a comprehensive article on his diagnosis and treatment in the May 13, 1996 issue of Fortune.

HDR is similar to conventional brachytherapy in that radioactive seeds are involved, but in this case the highly radioactive seeds are *temporarily* inserted in the prostate. This is repeated several times over a 48-hour period under local anesthesia. The seeds are finally removed, and then the patient typically undergoes several weeks of EBRT.

The Fortune article was four years old at the time, so I boldly decided to try contacting Mr. Grove to see what information I could gather from his experience. I called Intel corporate headquarters in Santa Clara, California and asked for Mr. Grove's office. His secretary ran interference and asked about the nature of my call. I told her my story, and said that I had a few questions for Mr. Grove. She suggested I e-mail him and gave me his e-mail address.

In my first e-mail, I indicated that I understood he is a high profile person, and that I would not reveal to others any personal or potentially embarrassing information that he shared with me. I listed several questions on the e-mail, including some very personal questions about the common side effects of the treatment.

His response was prompt, and surprisingly frank and detailed. I had more questions, so I sent more e-mails. He answered all my questions frankly and honestly.

As far as I know, Andy Grove is still cancer free, ten years after his treatment.

I continued my research into this form of treatment by tracking down and interviewing men who had chosen the brachytherapy option.   I spoke with a few "conventional" brachytherapy patients, but was unable to track down any others who had chosen the high dose option. I suspect it's because HDBT is not in wide use.

Two interesting anecdotes came out of my interviews with brachytherapy patients. The first involved a lawyer from New York. I received his name from one of his acquaintances. The lawyer agreed to speak with me on the condition that I keep his name confidential. I agreed and asked why. He told me that he was recently divorced and had two children and a new girlfriend. He told none of them of his diagnosis. He didn't want to frighten his kids or scare away his girlfriend. He also did not want his law firm partners to know.

After he was diagnosed, he conducted his research and chose brachytherapy. Secretly, he scheduled his seed implant treatment for a Friday afternoon and was back to work on the following Monday. When I spoke with him, which was two years later, his family, friends, and partners were unaware of his diagnosis and treatment.

Certainly, if someone can "bounce back" so quickly following a valid, proven treatment for prostate cancer, it was something that warranted serious consideration.

While I was doing my research, I received a call from a gentleman who heard I was evaluating prostate cancer treatment alternatives, and that I was interviewing former patients.   He happened to be an attorney as well, and was primarily focused on brachytherapy because of the minimal disruption to his lifestyle. I brought him up to date on my findings.

He asked if I could provide him the names of those I interviewed who had chosen brachytherapy. I gave him five names, and told him that I had a sixth name, a very well-informed gentleman who was a New York attorney, who asked me to keep his information confidential. He pleaded with me to get permission to talk with this gentleman. So I e-mailed the first lawyer, gave him the name, address, phone number, and e-mail address of the second lawyer, and encouraged him to call.

A week went by, and I received an e-mail from the first lawyer. He told me that coincidentally, the lawyer I referred to him was on the opposite side of a major legal battle on a very contentious case. However, under the circumstances, he called the second lawyer, shared his story, offered advice, and the two became friends – outside the courtroom. This certainly dispels one myth. Lawyers do have a heart – at least sometimes.

The one troubling thing my interviews of former brachytherapy patients revealed was lack of bladder control following treatment. About one in five reported varying levels of incontinence.

I concluded from my research that brachytherapy was a sound and viable treatment choice with its own unique set of advantages and disadvantages. And, if I were to go this route, my most important job was going to be to pick the right physician.

4. PROTON TREATMENT

Technically speaking, proton therapy is a form of external beam radiation therapy. But there are so many differences with this technology, due to the unique nature of the proton particle, that I felt it should be discussed separately.

As mentioned earlier, it is a widely known fact that radiation kills cancer. The more common form of radiation uses photons (X-rays) to attack the cancer. Photons begin to do their damage the instant they contact the body, and they give up that energy as they penetrate the body on the way to the tumor. After the photon radiation reaches the tumor, it continues to pass through the body, losing energy while continuing to pass through healthy cells as it exits the body.

Protons are sub-atomic particles, yet they are the largest particles in the atom. As such, they possess a unique characteristic called the *Bragg Peak*. This Bragg Peak refers to the proton beam's ability to pass into the body at high speed, travel to the location of a tumor deep within the body, and then release the bulk of its cancer-killing energy. Once the energy is released at the tumor site, there is *no* exit dose, and therefore, *no* radiation exposure to healthy tissue and organs on the far side of the tumor. This is a *major* difference from conventional photon/X-ray radiation, including IMRT, which dumps the *bulk* of its radiation energy on healthy tissue.

Technologies have been developed that allow the proton beam to be precisely shaped in three dimensions, and delivered to a site – such as the prostate – with extreme precision. One might look at conventional photon radiation as "carpet bombing" which does widespread damage around a target site. Proton radiation on the other hand is more like a "smart bomb" that precisely targets the tumor site while doing minimal collateral damage to nearby healthy organs and tissue. *This one factor is extremely important when it comes to potential side effects and "quality of life" issues following treatment.*

Since this form of radiation is so precisely targeted, the patient must be placed in the exact same position for each treatment. Customized devices must be designed and built for each patient to allow the proton radiation to conform, three-dimensionally, to the target site.

In order to receive this treatment, one must have a custom fit immobilization pod, a half-pipe-shaped device that is used to precisely position the patient daily for the eight weeks of treatment. A CT Scan is then done in order to produce a three dimensional image of the prostate and surrounding area. This information is used to plan the treatment protocol.

Treatment begins with the insertion of a small balloon-type device in the rectum, which is filled with a small amount of water. The balloon serves two purposes: it ensures the bulk of the rectal wall is out of range of the radiation beam, and it helps to immobilize the prostate.

The patient lies in the pod and is positioned in the center of a specially designed, 100 ton, three-story tall gantry. The customized focusing devices are attached to the machinery in the gantry, and the beam is delivered.

The entire treatment is painless and takes about one minute a day; however, preparation and safety protocols extend the total time in the treatment room to about 15 minutes.

Advantages of Proton Treatment:

- Cure rates are comparable to surgery and radiation.
- No hospitalization is required; treatment is done on an outpatient basis.
- It is noninvasive; there is no pain, no blood loss, no trauma, and zero recuperation time.
- Incontinence from this procedure is practically unheard of. The reported statistic is significantly less than 1%.

- Because of the unique characteristic of the proton particle (Bragg Peak), the tumor area can be more precisely targeted and therefore there is less collateral damage and fewer side effects, including fewer reported cases of impotence.

Disadvantages of Proton Treatment:

- Requires 8 weeks of treatment, five days a week
- Approximately 35% of the men treated report some changes in sexual potency.
- More expensive than other options. A small number of medical insurance providers still refuse to reimburse for proton therapy, resulting in some patients having to pay out of pocket. (See Chapter 14 on medical insurance)

One last point on proton treatment: All the statistics seem to verify that proton treatment cure rates are at *least* as good as the "gold standard," surgery. Ten year studies published in the International Journal of Radiation Oncology, Biology and Physics (Vol. 59, No. 2, pp 348-352, 2004) confirm this. My research convinced me that I could possibly expect even *better* results from proton therapy. Why? Because the routine procedure involved targeting the prostate, the capsule, the local seminal vesicles plus an extra 12-millimeter (half inch) margin. This margin is typically greater than the margin removed during surgery, and in all likelihood treats microscopic cancer cells that surgery might have missed. Further, the above studies were conducted on patients who received lower doses of proton radiation than is given today. Recent dose escalation clinical trials have resulted in higher allowable proton levels delivered to the tumor volume. One would expect cure rates to improve as more cancer-killing radiation finds its target. I suspect future studies will confirm this.

5. CRYOSURGERY

Cryosurgery – or Cryoablation – involves the controlled freezing of the prostate gland in order to destroy the cancerous cells. Studies dating back to the 1960s showed this technique worked, but complications frequently arose due to the difficulty in precisely monitoring and controlling the freezing process. Modern techniques have reportedly improved delivery techniques and minimized complications.

Patients often go on a three to six month hormone therapy program to shrink the prostate prior to treatment.

Either general or spinal anesthesia is administered and then needle punctures are made in the perineum – the area between the rectum and scrotum. Cryo probes are then inserted to freeze the prostate. Multiple thermocouples or temperature measuring devices are inserted to monitor the freezing process. A warming device is also inserted to protect the urethra. Two freezing cycles are performed and a catheter is then inserted to allow the bladder to be drained.

The procedure takes only a few hours and the patient is usually released the following day. The catheter must remain in place for about three weeks.

This technology is still relatively new and there is not a large patient population from which to draw statistics. Overall, results have been promising.

Advantages of Cryosurgery:

- Minimally invasive.
- Comparable cure rates to other options.
- Low cost.
- Quick recovery/recuperation.
- Other traditional options are available if this treatment fails.

Disadvantages of Cryosurgery:

- Limited database; only a small number of patients have been treated.
- Impotence reported in 85% of the cases, with only a small number of these regaining even partial potency.
- Incontinence rates are higher than with the other options and seem to vary, depending on the practitioner administering the treatment.
- Other urinary system complications are possible.

6. HORMONE ABLATION THERAPY

Hormone Ablation Therapy, or HAT, is also known as Androgen Deprivation Therapy, ADT. The term Ablation means deprivation, and this therapy is all about shutting down the male sex hormones (androgens) which are known to feed prostate cancer. The predominant androgen in the male is testosterone.

Often the treatment involves the use of a combination of drugs such as Lupron, Casodex and Zoladex. These drugs typically prevent the testicles, which produce the testosterone, from getting the message to do so. Unpleasant as it sounds, hormone therapy is a form of "temporary chemical castration." A common side effect is loss of libido.

Depriving the cancer of testosterone does not kill cancer; it merely retards the growth of cancer cells. Studies have shown that over time, the cancer cells can learn to thrive without their source of testosterone. For this reason, some doctors prescribe "intermittent hormonal therapy." This treatment, as the term suggests, involves the cycling on and off of hormone therapy over differing periods of time, depending on such measurements as PSA and testosterone level. The intent here is to "hold down" the cancer while preventing the cancer cells from becoming "refractory," or immune to hormone therapy.

Doctors have used hormone therapy for years to shrink prostates and large tumors prior to using other treatments for dealing with the prostate cancer. They have also used hormone therapy in conjunction with other treatments (e.g. surgery or radiation), especially for moderate to advanced prostate cancers.

Some medical institutions have recently begun studies using hormone therapy alone for early and mid stage prostate cancers. Results are reported to be promising.

Surgical removal of the testicles (called orchiectomy or castration) is another way of shutting down testosterone production of testosterone. This procedure is occasionally performed on patients with advanced prostate cancer.

Advantages of Hormone Therapy:

- Non invasive; no trauma; no blood loss; no hospitalization required.
- It can halt the growth of cancer while other options are being evaluated.
- Used as a "salvage" technique when other options fail.

Disadvantages of Hormone Therapy:

- Generally not considered a "cure," but a temporary measure to suppress cancer growth.
- Side effects: Loss of libido, hot flashes, weight gain, breast enlargement, depression, fatigue, reduction in genital size, and reduction in muscle and bone mass.

7. WATCHFUL WAITING

This is also called "Active Surveillance," and is a viable alternative for certain patients.

Watchful Waiting may be considered if you have very early stage prostate cancer with minimal PSA velocity, and you are at an age at which the predicted cancer growth would not typically produce any debilitating symptoms.

An individual with a 4.5 PSA, who has had a 20 sample biopsy, with cancer showing up in only 1 sample, with a 2+3=5 Gleason score, would be considered early stage. One must remember, however, that the biopsy is only a *sampling* process, and it may have missed an area of more aggressive cancer.

Typically, a patient who is on a watchful waiting program would monitor PSA closely, perhaps every three months at first, shifting to every six months if PSA is relatively stable over time.

Older men with moderate stage prostate cancer may also consider watchful waiting, particularly if their PSA velocity is such that debilitating symptoms would not be predicted during his lifetime.

Advantages of Watchful Waiting:

- The patient avoids the pain, trauma, potential blood loss, infection, and complications from anesthesia, which are possible from the surgical option.
- He avoids the invasiveness of seeds and cryosurgery, and inconvenience of the various radiation options.
- Side effects from any of the major treatment options are virtually eliminated, so bladder control and sexual potency are maintained.

Disadvantages of Watchful Waiting:

- Psychologically, the patient knows there is cancer growing in the prostate with no action being taken to destroy it. Some are uncomfortable living under these conditions.
- The cancer may grow, spread beyond the prostate, limiting treatment options in the future.

An Important Milestone is Reached

I remember sitting in my home office, reflecting on all I had learned so far – from books, the Internet and my interviews. It struck me that I had achieved an important milestone, and fulfilled a promise I had made to myself two years earlier while standing next to my brother in the recovery room following his surgery.

That day, I made a promise to myself, that if/when I was diagnosed with prostate cancer, I would find an option that was less barbaric than surgery, and one that would result in less impact on my quality of life *after* treatment. I remember sitting in my office with my feet on the desk, a smug look on my face, and feeling great relief, realizing I had found *several* options that met these criteria.

I also remember wondering, "Why do so many men choose surgery, when just about all the other options afford them the *same* chance of a cure, but without the trauma, blood loss, and side effects associated with surgery?" The answer, I would later discover, is that many men don't take the time to do their homework. They typically choose the specialty practiced by the physician who diagnosed them – their urologist.

I have no doubt most urologists believe their treatment is best. But so do the radiation oncologists, brachytherapists, and cryotherapists . . . and for that matter, watchful waiting proponents, the homeopaths, and alternative medicine practitioners. So, it's up to the patient to do his due diligence and pick a treatment based on thorough analysis and a comprehensive evaluation of *all* the options. The treatment you choose may still fail, but at least you won't be second guessing yourself if you later learned there was another treatment option you would have chosen if you had known about it.

I truly had reached an important milestone. Surgery was off the table – pun intended.

CHAPTER 7

Proton Treatment is Beginning to Look More and More Attractive

"Our real blessings often appear to us in the shape of pains, losses and disappointments, but let us have patience and we soon shall see them in their proper figures."

-- Joseph Addison

Could This New Treatment be for Me?

The more I read and heard about proton therapy, the more it felt like the right choice for me. The benefits: no trauma, no pain, no discomfort, minimal radiation damage to surrounding organs and tissue, and . . . minimal, if any, side effects. Most important, the statistical cure rates were at least comparable with those of the "gold standard," surgery, as well as the other major treatment methods.

But, I still had some doubts and a lot of questions. This treatment procedure appeared to be relatively new. How many patients had been treated? How many had been cured? Were the claims of minimal side effects true? Was this procedure experimental? If so, would my insurance company pay for it?

Even if insurance paid for it, what about out of pocket cost for travel, car rental, and living expenses? And what about the inconvenience? The treatment would take eight weeks. In the fall of 2000, there was only one place in the world that offered this treatment: Loma Linda University Medical Center (LLUMC) in Southern California. I would have to relocate from Massachusetts to this unknown city for eight weeks, and possibly miss Thanksgiving and Christmas at home with my family.

And in the back of my mind was another burning question: If this treatment is so good, why isn't it offered all over the world?

The more I learned, it seemed, the more questions I had. And the more I learned about proton therapy, the more I *wanted* it to be right for me. But I had to be sure.

Questions for the Medical Center

Now I was getting anxious. I remember 'beating myself up' one day and thinking, "It's been four weeks since my diagnosis, and all I've accomplished is to rule out surgery." But was I really being fair to myself? No. I had learned volumes about the other major treatment options, and I was zeroing in on one that could be right for me – one that still seemed too good to be true. It was time to learn more about proton therapy.

I called 1-800-PROTONS, the Loma Linda University Medical Center (LLUMC) referral office. In contrast to my contacts with the other practitioners, the medical professionals at Loma Linda, promptly returned my calls and always had time to talk with me. The people I spoke with at the Referral Office were extremely caring, professional, and responsive.

I faxed them a list of questions, and the next day they faxed me the answers.

Q 1: Do you need to know the precise location of tumor(s) in order for this therapy to be successful? In my case, my urologist tells me that the cancer sites are microscopic and cannot be felt or seen by ultrasound.

A 1: In terms of knowing the precise location of the tumor, we know from the biopsy that it is in your prostate gland, and in all probability it's confined there. Our radiation treatment field would include the entire gland, plus the capsule, the proximal (local) seminal vesicles, plus an extra 12-millimeter margin.

Q 2: In my case, cancer was only seen in the left lobe of my prostate. Would you treat *just* the left lobe, or the entire prostate?

74

If you treat just the left lobe, how do you know there isn't cancer in the right lobe? The biopsy, after all is only a sample.

A 2: As stated in the previous answer, the entire prostate gland is treated to give us the best chance of destroying all the cancer cells.

Q 3: How do you protect my urethra, which runs through the middle of my prostate?

A 3: You are quite right; the urethra runs through the prostate and thus is in the radiation path. However, the urethra is surprisingly tolerant of radiation and it typically handles the radiation well. Occasionally there are temporary side effects such as burning during urination, and possibly spasms of the urethra. We have medications that can treat these symptoms, which typically subside after the treatment ends.

Q 4: I read that proton therapy is suited for "localized, solid tumors." Does this mean it is not suited for my early stage prostate cancer, which is microscopic and cannot be seen by ultrasound?

A-4: No. Proton therapy is highly suited for early stage prostate cancer such as yours. We have a well-defined target – the prostate gland – even though we cannot see the cancer cells themselves.

Q 5: How many prostate cancer patients have been treated at Loma Linda? What are the statistics on cure rate, especially ranked by pretreatment PSA and Gleason score? Can you send me a copy of the statistics?

A 5: Yes, I have mailed you some published information on this subject.

Q 6: Before I travel to California I would like to speak with prostate cancer patients who have received treatment there. Can you give me some names and telephone numbers?

A 6: Yes, I will fax you a list of prior patients who are on a volunteer call list and are willing to speak with you.

Q 7: What are the typical side effects of this treatment? What would you expect in my case?

A 7: Side effects can include fatigue, urinary problems, impotence, possible increase in frequency of stools, rectal irritation and/or discomfort. The severity of these varies from person to person and depends on your health, present urinary symptoms (which I see in your case is none), and energy level going into treatment. Generally, most patients tolerate this treatment very well and report minimal side effects.

Q 8: It appears that proton therapy is only *sometimes* effective in killing cancer cells. See the following quotes. Am I misinterpreting these statements from Internet publications?

"While both normal and cancerous cells go through this repair process (after proton therapy treatment), a cancer cell's ability to repair itself is *frequently* inferior - - -"

"Damaging the DNA destroys specific cell functions, which *may* include the ability to divide or proliferate - - -"

"A cancer cell's ability to repair molecular injury is *frequently* inferior. As a result, cancer cells sustain *more permanent* damage and subsequent cell death than occurs in the normal cell population."

A 8: I think if you are interpreting these statements as being unique to proton beam treatment and its efficacy, then yes, that's probably a misinterpretation. No cancer therapy is 100% effective, unfortunately. That is also true for surgery, all forms of radiation, chemotherapy, etc. The sentences you quote refer to cancer cells in general, and so they use words like "frequently," "may," etc. Almost any cell in the body can lose its ability to regulate its growth normally and become cancerous, and as they start out as different kinds of cells (i.e. lung cells, glandular cells, brain cells, etc.) they don't all behave exactly the same way. This

76

in turn means that they can respond to treatments differently. Some respond to chemotherapy very well, some do not. Some respond better to radiation than others. We know that the proton beam can kill cancer in the prostate. But we can never be absolutely sure that none of those cells has escaped and traveled to another part of the body. As compared to other forms of cancer that are considered to be aggressive and metastasize readily, prostate cancer is relatively slow growing.

Q 9: Is my specific case a good fit for Loma Linda PT therapy?

A 9: Yes, your cancer is considered early stage. Early stage cancers typically have the best outcomes.

Q 10: Is surgery no longer an option if proton therapy fails?

A 10: Many urologists will not do surgery on someone who has had radiation therapy for prostate cancer, but some specialists can and will do this procedure. But when radiation therapy fails, it usually fails because the cancer had previously moved outside the field that was treated. If this is the case, why consider surgery to remove the gland? There are other aspects of this issue that would best be discussed with your doctor if you come in for a consult.

Q 11: How much total time should I expect to spend at Loma Linda including pre-testing and preparations?

A 11: The treatment is 8 weeks in duration, Monday through Friday, daily treatments. A CT scan of your pelvis will be done to be used to plan your treatment and it takes about 1 to 2 weeks to start treatment once that CT is done.

Q 12: Can you tell me about living arrangements and costs?

A 12: There are numerous alternatives available to you. I will send you this information in the mail.

Q 13: Based on what you have seen of my specific case and considering all the treatment options available to me, what treatment option would you select if you were in my shoes?

A 13: That decision is, of course, up to you. Even though I'm not a man, I think I can understand not wanting to have to live with some of the possible side effects of prostate cancer treatment. Our treatment is as effective as surgery or conventional radiation and with generally fewer side effects.

Q 14: In my case, what is the degree of urgency for treatment? (ASAP, this month, this year, next year?)

A 14: This is hard to answer and best discussed with a physician. I would say that if you get treatment in a couple of months it should be fine. I think waiting a year would not be a wise thing to do.

Q 15: If I qualify, when could you take me?

A 15: We could schedule you for a consult in about a month.

I was satisfied with these answers, and within a few days I would have new ammunition. I would have data, which compared proton therapy with other treatment options. I was elated by their promise to send me the names of men who had received proton treatment. Talking with them, I knew, would be a major factor in making my decision.

As promised, the next day I received a fax with a list of 30 names, addresses, treatment dates, and phone numbers. This astounded me! For a month I had been struggling to get the names of men who had received various forms of treatment such as EBRT, brachytherapy, and cryosurgery, and met with considerable resistance. The response from the doctor's office was typically, "We need to respect the privacy of the patient and cannot give out names" (This was before today's strict HIPAA regulations on patient confidentiality). I told them, I didn't want to invade their privacy. I just wanted to talk with them about their experience of treatment, and they could do that anonymously, "Give them my number, have them call me," I pleaded. I had questions only someone on the "receiving end" of the treatment could answer.

The doctors and their nurses representing the other treatment options seemed "put off" by my request. They told me *they* could

78

answer all my questions, and there really wasn't any need for me to talk with their patients. The more they resisted, the more I persisted.

I have always believed that a *salesman* will tell you almost anything to make the sale. It's the *customer* who will give you the *real* story about a product or service. He/she has nothing to gain or lose by being totally honest. In all my business dealings, I had relied heavily on customer satisfaction when choosing a vendor for a product or service. I also relied heavily on reference checks when hiring key people to work for me – just one more way of checking with a former 'customer.'

When I received the Loma Linda list of former proton patients, I established a plan. This was to call every man on the list, beginning with those who were treated in the early 1990s. I prepared a list of questions, and typed up a survey sheet where I would collect 22 pieces of data on every man I spoke with (remember, I'm a recovering engineer!). I planned to ask each his age, cancer stage (PSA, Gleason score, T score), when they were treated, short and long-term side effects, and much more.

Then the thought occurred to me, "How do I know these folks from Loma Linda didn't 'stack the deck?' They probably sent me a list of their success cases. How could I be sure I would be speaking with a representative group of former patients?" The solution to this dilemma was simple. As part of my survey, I would ask each man to give me the names of two patients he met while in treatment. If they spent eight weeks in that small town, surely they would have developed relationships with other proton patients.

I remember sleeping well that night, knowing that I was about to add much to my knowledge base in the coming days.

My Survey

Following is the survey form I used for my interviews with former proton patients.

Name: _____ Phone: _____ Date: _____

Age when treated? _____ Current Age: _____ Treatment End Date: _____

Cancer stage (T1, T2, etc.): __ Palpable Tumor by DRE? ___Gleason Score: _____

Name of Insurance Company: _____ Did they pay? _____

Any side effects (short term, long term)?_____
_____

Current condition (PSA, symptoms)?_____
_____

Any other form of treatment done (hormone, photon radiation, surgery)?_____
_____

What major factors influenced your decision to choose Proton? _____
_____
_____

What was your experience of LLUMC and the treatment process?_____
_____
_____

What was your urologist's reaction to your decision to choose Proton? _____
_____

Who was your doctor and case manager? Would you recommend them? _____
_____

Would you make the same decision again? _____

What other information can you give me to help me make my decision? _____
_____

Can you give me the names and phone numbers of two men you know who went through Proton treatment?_____
_____
_____

Survey Results

I was pleasantly surprised by the receptivity of the men I called, as well as their friendliness and willingness to share intimate details of their diagnosis, treatment and follow-up. I would later learn that men with prostate cancer feel a bonding, or sense of brotherhood, and generally go out of their way to help others facing the same challenges.

Several of the men on the list had moved or changed phone numbers and were unreachable, but I was able to contact twenty. Each happily answered all my questions, and gave me the names of others with whom they were treated. Over a six-day period I spoke with 56 former proton patients. And I had certainly bracketed my areas of interest: ages 51 to 84, PSAs 2.5 to 27, Gleason scores 4 to 9, stages T1c to T3 (A to C).

What did I learn from these interviews? Volumes! I had struck gold! Following is a summary of what I heard from these former Proton patients:

Side Effects

Most claimed that the side effects were minimal to non-existent. Eight men (14%) reported some occasional, minor rectal bleeding, which began several months after treatment ended. In six of the eight cases it had stopped. The other two reported it was minimal and they expected it to go away. I later learned that temporary, minor rectal bleeding is not uncommon with radiation treatment. It is a result of a phenomenon called radiation induced neovascularization. Healthy cells on the interior wall of the rectum that were exposed to some radiation – because of the 12 mm margin treated – typically repair themselves, forming new blood vessels. Occasionally these blood vessels 'leak' blood into the stool. This condition is usually temporary, painless, and it almost always goes away on its own.

A few of those I spoke with reported some urinary urgency or urinary burning during the later stages of treatment, which subsided after treatment ended.

Most reported normal sex lives, albeit with significantly less ejaculate (all treatment options reduce or eliminate ejaculate, usually with no impact on sexual performance or pleasure).

Those, with more advanced cancers, who were on adjunct hormone therapy were experiencing a loss of libido, which they said they "hoped" was temporary. One gentleman who had stopped hormone therapy admitted to not regaining sexual function. Twelve (21%) felt their sexual potency had diminished somewhat following proton treatment. When questioned further, the common theme was more difficulty achieving erections, and/or less firmness with erections. One respondent offered that, "Sex has definitely changed for me. I'm down to only twice a week! But my age might have something to do with it. I was 84 last month."

Most of those with diminished potency who tried Erectile Dysfunction medications reported positive results.

None of the 56 reported having any problems with incontinence. Let me repeat. Not a single person reported having *any* problems with bladder control. This was my number one concern. I was feeling better about proton treatment.

Current PSA

Every person I spoke with felt he was in a much better space for having chosen proton treatment. PSAs were dramatically reduced in every case. All but one reported PSAs below 1.0. Those treated three or more years earlier felt they had reached their PSA nadir (low point). Several indicated their PSAs were "still coming down."

Other Treatments They Received

About a third of the men I spoke with were given some additional form of treatment – photon radiation and/or hormone therapy. Photon radiation was prescribed, in addition to proton therapy, for those whose cancers might have progressed beyond the prostate gland as indicated by DRE, high PSA, and/or high Gleason score. Photon radiation is used to treat the entire prostate bed including lymph nodes. Typically, the same total amount of radiation is delivered, but it is split between the two forms.

Hormone treatment in conjunction with proton or proton/photon was common for men with very large prostates and/or advanced cancers.

Temporary side effects from hormones included hot flashes, loss of sexual desire, and occasionally enlarged breasts. Photon radiation occasionally resulted in temporary fatigue. Other than fatigue, those who were treated with proton and photon did not seem to experience any more severe side effects than those treated with proton alone.

Major Factors Influencing Their Decision

Surprisingly, a large percentage of the men I spoke with were scientists, engineers, physicists, doctors, lawyers, educators, and business leaders. They all seemed to have analytical minds, and an interest and ability to review, digest, and understand technical information.

They all did their homework and researched the alternatives. None blindly accepted their urologist's initial recommendation, which in almost every case was surgery. All were convinced that radiation kills cancer; that proton therapy is the most advanced and precise form of radiation therapy; that their chance of a cure with proton therapy was at least as good as other standard treatments; and that side effects with protons were minimal, giving them the best chance of a high quality of life after treatment.

Their Experience of LLUMC and the Treatment Process

If there were any doubts in their minds as to the efficacy of the treatment or the medical professionals at the hospital, they were quickly dispelled when they visited the Proton Treatment Facility at Loma Linda University Medical Center and met with the staff. Every respondent expressed superlatives about the doctors, case managers, technicians, and support staff. It sounded too good to be true.

Urologists' Reaction

Most of the men I spoke with told me their urologists were opposed to their choosing proton treatment. Their doctors described the treatment as "experimental, investigational, early stage, unproven, or dangerous." Several urologists told their patients to "find yourself another doctor if you do proton treatment." A few were more open minded and offered their best wishes. Only one urologist indicated he knew of proton therapy, that it was a viable alternative, and he supported the decision.

Doctor and Case Manager

The responses here were actually humorous and enlightening: *"My doctor was Carl Rossi. He's been there the longest, wrote most of the papers, and is clearly the best one on the faculty. Make sure you choose him."*

"Dr. Jabola was my physician. You must make sure you get him. He's the best one there."

"Dr. Bush is the number one guy. Insist on having him as your physician."

"Richard Levy is the one who treated me. Look no further. You won't find a finer doctor than he."

"Don't accept anyone other than Dr. Yonemoto. He really knows his stuff, and he really takes care of his patients. He's the one you want."

This happened over and over, and I learned something, that was confirmed later when I went through treatment: All the physicians at LLUMC are superb. They all are brilliant physicians/physicists, who treat their patients in the finest tradition of the LLUMC Mission Statement, "To Make Man Whole."

I later learned something else about proton therapy that sets it apart from surgery and brachytherapy. *Proton therapy is not practitioner dependent*. It really didn't matter which doctor you chose at Loma Linda. The procedures are all documented and well established. And, following the initial CT scan, the customized treatment protocol is reviewed with a team of physicians, dosimetrists and physicists. Every single case is reviewed by a *team* of competent professionals.

Cancer Recurrence

One of the men I interviewed reported his cancer had returned. It is interesting to note that he was on the original call list I received from Loma Linda, not one I had found through my survey. He reported that his PSA began to rise three years after treatment ended, and that a biopsy of his prostate detected no cancer. He said that prior to treatment his cancer had moved outside the area treated and the proton therapy did its job killing the cancer in his prostate. He told me the quality of his life had not changed one bit since he was treated; he had no regrets for having chosen proton therapy; and he highly recommended it to me. He was now in the process of researching salvage treatment options and was optimistic about the future.

Would You Make the Same Decision Again?

This question received an unequivocal and resounding *yes* from every respondent.

But What About Andy Grove?

This all seemed too good to be true. But something was still troubling me. If proton therapy is this good, then why didn't Andy Grove choose it when he was treated in the mid 90s? He was a wealthy business leader who could have had any treatment at any medical institution in the world. Why didn't he choose proton? I speculated that it was because he was a busy executive and couldn't afford to be away from his office for eight weeks.

To answer this question, I sent him one last e-mail and asked, "Mr. Grove, I have been researching treatment options, and I am leaning toward Proton Beam Therapy at Loma Linda University Medial Center. In your position, you could have chosen any treatment, anywhere in the world. Proton therapy appears to me to be the best option available by a wide margin. Why didn't you choose it?"

His answer was right to the point, "Bob, I had never heard of proton beam therapy, so it was never a treatment I considered."

CHAPTER 8

My Treatment Decision

Life consists not in holding good cards, but in playing those you hold, well.

-- Josh Billings

The Value of Talking with Other Men

Looking back at all my efforts in researching the alternatives, clearly the greatest value for me was in speaking with men who had chosen each of the treatment options. They filled in all the missing pieces, most of which I would never have found on the Internet or in the countless books and articles that have been written on prostate cancer.

Tip: Before making your treatment choice, speak with several men who have had each form of treatment you are considering. Their personal experience will be invaluable to you in making the decision that is best for you.

The Process of Elimination

I was clearly leaning toward proton therapy at Loma Linda, but I had to be sure. Sometimes it pays to be an anal retentive, obsessive compulsive, recovering engineer.

I quickly ruled out Watchful Waiting. I was too young and had too many years for the cancer to grow and metastasize, and my PSA had been rising rapidly during the past two years. Why should I give this thing growing inside me a chance to migrate beyond the gland and move into my lymph nodes, eventually metastasizing and traveling to the rest of my body? No, Watchful Waiting was not for me.

Cryoablation was relatively new, and there were minimal statistics on which to base a decision. I also had difficulty finding people to talk with who had received this treatment. And, what little I had heard about side effects, particularly urinary incontinence, frightened me.

I couldn't think of one valid reason for keeping Radical Prostatectomy on the "short list." It is major surgery; it is a complex and bloody procedure; side effects are many, and are more severe than the alternatives; results are extremely practitioner dependent; and 0.5% of the patients die on the operating table. It only works if the cancer is totally confined to the prostate, whereas most of the other treatments provide the added benefit of treating a certain "margin" around the prostate. Surgery was definitely off the list, and I felt a huge weight lifted off my shoulders.

Laparoscopic radical prostatectomy was brand new in 2000, and I couldn't find any published information on the subject. I have since learned that, while patients recover more quickly from this type of surgery, the complications and side effects are essentially the same as open surgery. So it would still be off my list.

This left brachytherapy, 3D-Conformal External Beam Radiation Therapy (3D-CRT), IMRT, and proton treatment.

I continued to search the Internet, seek out new books, and interview former patients. Facts began to emerge that shed some new light on brachytherapy. Nineteen percent of the seeds implanted in the prostate tend to dislodge and migrate to different parts of the body. Some pass through the urethra and leave the body with the urine; others find their way to the lungs. I realized that the half-life of the radiation in these seeds was very short. Nevertheless, the thought of having even low-level radioactive seeds settling in my lungs was disconcerting.

I continued my interviews with former patients representing the remaining treatment options and learned of two cases of incontinence connected with seed implants. One attorney, who had chosen seeds, told me he carried two briefcases – one with his legal material and the other full of diapers. He said he couldn't sit through a meeting longer than one hour without having to change his diaper. This bothered me even more than the issue of seed migration.

There also appeared to be a higher incidence of bladder neck stricture and urinary tract blockage with seeds. I assumed that was due to the significantly higher dose of radiation to the urethra, which passes through the center of the prostate.

Earlier I mentioned that success with brachytherapy was extremely practitioner dependent. I was now learning that in addition to killing the cancer, treatment success is also measured in terms of factors such as seed migration.

The few 'premier' brachytherapy specialists were practically untouchable. I attempted to make an appointment with one, and was told it would be several months before I could see him. Even then I might find he wouldn't take me as a patient, or I might be "diverted" to one of his associates.

For all the above reasons, I took brachytherapy off the list, and decided I would only reconsider seed if I could have the procedure done by Dr. John Blasko at the Seattle Prostate Institute.

The more I looked into 3D-CRT, the more I was discovering its use to be in conjunction with other treatments such as surgery, hormones, or proton. It seemed that conformal photon (X-ray) radiation with its broad range, "shot gun" or "carpet bomb" delivery of radiation was good for "mopping up" around the tumor site, especially if the cancer was more advanced and there was a high probability it had escaped the gland. But I was convinced this option carried with it a much higher probability of undesirable side effects.

IMRT made a lot of sense and really had my interest, but I saw two negatives. First, in 2000 it was still relatively new. There was practically no data available on this option, and I was having great difficulty finding former IMRT patients to interview. And second, IMRT still used photon radiation, and that meant a higher probability of collateral damage – side effects.

Proton treatment was looking better and better.

Nick DeWolf

There is something about prostate cancer that makes a fraternity out of its victims. Once I broke through the resistance of the doctors, I found patients were much more than willing to share information. All along the way, I met countless former patients who gave generously of their time to tell me their story and help me in my decision making process. None was more helpful than Nick DeWolf.

Nick was diagnosed in 1996 and chose a combination Proton/Photon treatment at Loma Linda. Before making his decision, he did exhaustive research into the alternatives and examined each technology in great detail. As co-founder of Teradyne and now a retired "technocrat," Nick was comfortable wallowing in such terms as atoms, protons, photons, rads, cobalt-gray, ionization, and apoptosis.

As a service to his fellow man, Nick developed a comprehensive website, www.protons.com, where he methodically chronicled his journey.

I discovered Nick's website one Sunday afternoon while surfing the Internet and I read everything he wrote, explored every link, and studied every graph. One thing in particular, caught my attention – his "Decision Matrix."

Here, Nick prepared his own somewhat subjective analysis of the four options he was considering: Proton, EBRT, Surgery, and Surgery plus X-ray. He identified all the factors he considered in his decision making process, which included such things as probability of a cure, convenience, and short and long term side effects. Some factors were rated based on probabilities of occurrence; other factors were given weighted values, and then scored based on his research.

With Nick's permission, I have reproduced his Decision Matrix here in Figure 8-1, along with his introduction.

Here is a Matrix that may assist you in deciding your treatment choice. Each factor was weighted by its maximum (subjective importance) and my judgment (subjective) of my odds. Bigger values mean worse results. Other patients would alter the values widely, but this reasoning made my choice very easy.

		Radiation		Surgery	
		Proton	**X-ray**		
Include X-ray phase 2?	-	Yes	Yes	No	Yes
Hormone Adjuvant (months)		No	3	4-6	4-6
Days away from home	-	60	60	8	70
Days to ¾ recovery		0	0	80	80
Cost (relative)		30	15	15	25
Scoring	**Max**	**G u e s t i m a t i o n s**			
Likelihood of recurrence	500	50	100	200	50
Likelihood of induced cancer	100	5	10	0	10
Operating room traumas	100	0	0	50	50
Subtotal:	700	55	110	250	110
Short term side effects					
Pain	50	0	0	20	20
Incontinence	15	0	5	15	15
Frequency of urination	15	5	10	15	15
Diarrhea	15	5	10	10	15
Exhaustion	40	10	10	20	25
Loss of Sexual Pleasure	25	5	5	15	15
Erectile Impotence	15	4	8	10	15
Inconvenience	25	10	10	5	12
Subtotal:	**200**	**39**	**58**	**110**	**132**
Longer term side effects					
Rectal & bladder damage	100	6	12	10	20
Pain	250	0	4	60	60
Incontinence	100	4	8	20	25
Frequency of urination	50	4	6	15	20
Diarrhea	100	4	6	10	15
Exhaustion	200	5	6	50	50
Loss of sexual pleasure	150	10	15	80	80
Erectile impotence	40	4	8	20	20
Infertility	10	3	3	10	10
Inconvenience	100	5	5	20	30
Subtotal	**1100**	**45**	**73**	**290**	**325**
Grand Total	**2000**	**139**	**241**	**650**	**567**
	Worst	Proton	X-rays	Surgery	

This approach really resonated with me. It was 9:00 PM when I finished exploring Nick's site. Since he kindly provided a link with his e-mail address and an offer to respond to questions, I sent him an e-mail and asked if I could talk with him personally.

At 10:00 PM my phone rang. It was Nick DeWolf. We spoke for two hours. I was impressed with his intellect and his candor. He graciously answered all my questions and offered to make himself available at any time if I had more questions or just wanted to talk. I remember hanging up the phone that night, making a promise that if I beat this disease, I would do everything I could to help prostate cancer patients the way Nick DeWolf helped me.

Time to Visit Loma Linda

Although I was now about 90% sure I wanted to do proton, I hadn't made up my mind. What was it going to take? What would convince me that proton treatment was the best option? After wrestling with these questions for a while, the answer became obvious. I had to see, feel and touch proton therapy. I had to visit the facility, look at the equipment, and speak with the people who practiced this technology.

During the dozens of hours of patient interviews, I came across two gentlemen who had made their mark at Loma Linda. They had endeared themselves with doctors and staff with their charm, their humor, and the dozens of boxes of doughnuts they brought to the Proton Treatment Center each morning for the radiation therapists.

Both were on the patient call list that the hospital sent me. So I called Joe Gazzola and Joe Praught, and asked for an introduction to Dr. Carl Rossi, the man whose name appeared on most of the proton therapy technical publications, the radiation oncologist who had been there from the day the Proton Treatment Center opened. The 'two Joes' told me that the way to reach Dr. Rossi was through his Nurse/Case Manager, an extraordinary lady named Sharon Hoyle. I would later give her the pseudonym, "Florence Nightingale."

I called Sharon, introduced myself as a friend of 'the two Joes,' and asked for her assistance in seeing Dr. Rossi. Sharon arranged the appointment and offered one other suggestion. As long as I was making the trip across country, why not plan to have my CT Scan and custom immobilization pod fabricated on the same visit? This would save me two to four weeks and another cross-country trip, if I decided to choose the treatment (she knew I would). If I decided *not* to do the treatment, I would have to pay for these things out of pocket. I agreed.

I flew to Ontario airport in California, rented a car, and stayed at a local motel that offered discounts to Loma Linda patients. The next morning I drove to the medical center and was instantly overwhelmed by its size. The San Bernardino valley sits between two mountain ranges, and most of the land in the valley is flat. Houses and commercial buildings are generally one to three story buildings. Towering above everything else in the valley was the Loma Linda University Medical Center (LLUMC).

All the buildings were white and were surrounded by support buildings, student and staff dormitories, and a chapel. The grounds and parking areas were meticulously maintained. Despite the desert climate, the grounds were lush with green grass and flowers. A helicopter was landing on the roof as I searched for a parking space in one of their huge parking lots (I later learned that LLUMC is a major trauma center for southern California and Medivac helicopters routinely shuttle patients in from hundreds of miles away.).

First Impressions

High on a tower over the main entrance of the hospital was a large cross and the words, "Loma Linda University Medical Center a Seventh-day Adventist Institution." I am not an overly religious person, and I am not an Adventist, but seeing the cross and reading those words gave me an instant feeling of peace and comfort.

A security officer greeted me as I approached the front door, and I was warmly welcomed by the receptionist at the main desk, given a visitor's pass, and directed to the Proton Treatment Center.

To my surprise, the unit was three stories beneath the earth and directly under the children's hospital. I later learned that for safety reasons, construction was done beneath the earth, and the critical systems were surrounded by fourteen-foot thick concrete and steel walls.

Sharon Hoyle was there to welcome me, take down some information, put me completely at ease, and usher me in to Dr. Rossi's office. I was struck by Dr. Rossi's apparent youth. This expert in the field, the man who had been helping to pioneer this technique since 1990 and had published so many articles on the subject, appeared to be about thirty-five years old. I remember thinking, "This guy could be my son!"

I gave Dr. Rossi my paperwork, which included my medical history and pathology reports, and we discussed my case in great detail. He answered all my questions clearly, concisely, and honestly. I was impressed with his knowledge, his intellect, his manner, his humility, and the amount of uninterrupted time he gave me.

Orientation Tour

Next I was introduced to Gerry Troy, a social worker who was head of Patient Services for the Proton Center. Gerry conducted a two-hour tour of the facility, explaining the systems and technology. I remember thinking, "How can a 'shrink' be this knowledgeable about the technology of proton treatment?" 'Gerry-the-shrink' would later become a good friend.

Gerry explained in great detail how the proton particle was extracted from hydrogen gas, then introduced to the accelerator, speeded-up in a particle accelerator, called a synchrotron, and delivered to the treatment rooms. He also explained how the prostate was imaged three dimensionally by the CT Scan; how the dosimetrists, physicists and radiation oncologists custom tailor a treatment plan for each patient; and how focusing devices, called apertures and boluses were constructed for each patient, in order to conform the proton beam precisely to the target area.

He also showed us where and how the immobilization pod was made to ensure each patient is placed in exactly the same position every day for treatment. And, he explained how a small water-filled balloon was used to protect the rectum during the daily treatments. This point caught my attention.

Gerry then brought us three floors down to the treatment areas. There I saw three giant gantries and a "fixed beam" room. Each Gantry was three stories high, consisting of more than 100 tons of steel and concrete, and designed to rotate within extremely tight tolerances around the patient being treated.

A few days earlier, I wasn't sure what to expect as I conjured up images from my home in Massachusetts. But what I saw was nothing like what I expected. This was not some 'fly by night' Frankenstein laboratory, with mad scientists scurrying about. What I saw was a 'star wars' type, ultra modern, super clean facility, staffed by competent professionals.

That evening I attended one of the weekly Wednesday night support group meetings. This popular meeting is attended by prospective patients (like myself), current patients, former patients, and others. New patients, called 'Newbies,' share stories of how they discovered proton therapy. Patients who are completing treatment, called 'Graduates,' talk about their eight-week odyssey, usually in humorous terms, often accompanied by poetry, music, or comedy skits. Visiting Graduates, called 'Alumni,' often return to report how they are doing months or years after treatment.

The meeting was scheduled to begin at 5:30 PM. I arrived at 5:15 PM and thought I was in the wrong place. The hallway outside the meeting room was jammed with high spirited people who were lined up for sandwiches, cookies, and fruit drinks. Most of the chairs in the meeting room were occupied, and the remaining ones were disappearing fast. Everyone was smiling, some were laughing, and the atmosphere was festive. It felt like I had walked in on a group of people who had won the lottery. In a way I had.

Gerry Troy called the meeting to order. It took a full five minutes to quiet the crowd and then Gerry began to talk. Without any introduction, he said:

"A man from Texas, driving a Volkswagen Beetle, pulls up next to a guy in a Rolls Royce at a stop sign. Their windows are open and he yells at the guy in the Rolls, "Hey, you got a telephone in that Rolls?"

The guy in the Rolls replies: "Yes, of course I do."

"I got one too… see?" the Texan says.

"Uh, yes that's very nice."

"You got a fax machine too?" the Texan asks.

"Why, actually, yes I do."

"I do too! See, it's right here," brags the Texan.

The light is about to turn green and the man in the Beetle says:

"So, do you have a double bed in the back there?"

"NO! Do you?"

"Yep, got my double bed right in the back," the Texan replies.

The light turns and the Beetle takes off.

Well, the guy in the Rolls is not about to be one-upped, so he immediately goes to a customizing shop and orders them to put in a double bed on the back of the Rolls. About two weeks later, the job is finally done.

He picks up his car and drives all over town looking for the Volkswagen Beetle with the Texas plates. Finally, he finds it parked alongside the road, so he pulls his Rolls up next to it.

The windows on the Volkswagen are all fogged up and he feels somewhat awkward about it, but he gets out of his newly modified Rolls and taps on the foggy window of the Volkswagen.

The man in the Volkswagen finally opens a window and peeks out. The guy in the Rolls says, "Hey, remember me?"

"Yeah, I remember you," says the Texan. "What's up?"

"Check this out... I got a double bed installed in my Rolls."

The Texan exclaims: "YOU GOT ME OUT OF THE SHOWER TO TELL ME THAT?"

The room erupted in laughter. Then someone from the back of the room raised his hand and said, "I've got one better than that," and he proceeded to tell *his* joke. After two or three more, Gerry started to make his announcements. He ran down the list of upcoming activities including such things as, "*The Movers and Shakers* Group will meet on Thursday evening; the *Lunch Bunch* is going to *The Little Fisherman* on Friday; *Pod Partners* will meet on Monday at 3:30 PM; this week's restaurant tour will be at the Elk's Lodge; we have some free tickets for the *San Bernardino Symphony Orchestra* concert next week; the extended proton tour will be held at 10:00 on Saturday; tickets for the *Getty Museum* tour will be available on Friday; etc. The announcements went on for almost ten minutes.

Next, Gerry asked if there were any "Graduates" in the audience. About nine people raised their hands. Gerry called on them, one by one, and each gave a "graduation speech." The speeches included poems, songs, and humorous accounts of each patient's experience at Loma Linda. They had us laughing one minute and crying the next. All expressed their sincere appreciation to the staff for their extraordinary experience.

The fun continued. Next Gerry asked if there were any "Alumni" present. One by one, the Alumni stood up, recounting their journey since treatment. Alumni ranged from one man who had been treated for prostate cancer six years earlier and was doing "great," to a young woman who was successfully treated for an inoperable brain tumor a year ago. All were in good spirits and all thanked and praised LLUMC and the Lord for the "gift" they had been given. The spiritual atmosphere was evident in this room full of laughter and tears on that Wednesday evening.

Finally, Gerry asked for the "Newbies" to identify themselves. About 15 hands went up. Most were prostate cancer patients from the U.S., Europe and Australia. They reported their pretreatment PSAs and Gleason Scores and spoke about how they learned about proton treatment and Loma Linda. None seemed fearful or anxious about the treatment they were just beginning. Was I the only one in the room worried about this dreaded disease?

I looked at my watch; it was almost 8:00 PM. Where had the last 2 ½ hours gone? Why is everyone so cheery? The whole experience was beginning to feel surreal. "This room is filled with cancer patients," I thought, "How can they be so happy?"

I later learned that this meeting was just one of several psychosocial programs that LLUMC has instituted as part of their *Make Man Whole* mission.

Decision Made

While walking through the beautiful grounds of the Loma Linda University Medical Center the next day, and reflecting on the events since my arrival – the cross on the tower, the warm reception, the meeting with Dr. Rossi and Sharon Hoyle, the tour of the Proton Treatment Center, and the Wednesday night meeting – I made my decision. It was Proton Treatment for me!

I told Sharon Hoyle, my Case Manager, about my decision. She congratulated me and directed me to the team of people who would build my immobilization pod and do the CT scan.

The Pod, The Scan and My First Balloon

The immobilization pod is an approximately seven-foot long, half-tube constructed of PVC. I was asked to put on a one-size-fits-none hospital gown, often called a 'johnny.' This cover-up is often the butt of jokes – no pun intended – because of the embarrassment it causes patients. It's a short gown, tied in the back, often leaving one's backside exposed.

I donned the johnny and climbed into the pod, which was lined with a soft fabric. It felt a little like climbing into a coffin.

Then they gave me my first balloon. I cannot say that it was uncomfortable. I learned this device is an infant enema wand, a piece of hollow, semi-rigid rubber, the diameter of a pencil, about five inches long, with what appeared to be a condom stretched over it. The technician coated it with KY Jelly and inserted it in my rectum. Once in place, he 'inflated' it with four ounces of water.

As mentioned earlier, the function of the balloon is twofold. First it 'inflates' the colon to move the posterior (outside) wall of the rectum out of the range of the proton radiation. Secondly, it helps to immobilize the prostate by forcing it up against the pelvic bone. This ensures the prostate is always in the same position before daily radiation treatment. This day, they were doing it in order to prepare me for the CT scan.

While lying snugly in the pod, with my balloon firmly in place, the technician began pouring warm polyurethane between the PVC pod and the sheet on which I was lying. This produced a mold that conformed to my body and would essentially keep me motionless while I was being treated. I actually found it to be quite comfortable.

Now secure in my newly fabricated immobilization pod, I was wheeled into the CT Scan room. Over the next 20 minutes they took ninety-eight pictures or 'slices' of my anatomy in the prostate region. These pictures are used to produce a three dimensional "hologram" of my prostate which the oncologists, physicists and dosimetrists use to plan my treatment.

This information is also used to construct two custom-made focusing devices called an aperture and a bolus, which, along with a specific energy modulator, would be used together to conform the proton beam to the precise target area. This area, I was told included the prostate, the capsule surrounding the prostate, the nearby seminal vesicles and an extra half inch of margin around the whole 'package.'

With pod and CT Scan completed, I met with my Case Manager and requested a start date that would allow me to be home for Christmas. Despite the patient overload, Sharon made some adjustments and arranged a start date that would have me home by December 22nd. That is just one of the dozens of ways the people at LLUMC went out of their way to accommodate my needs and to make me feel like a special patient. I later learned from others that they all felt the same way.

Where Will We Live for Eight Weeks?

The next challenge I faced was finding a place to stay in the Loma Linda area for my two-month out-patient treatment period. Again the folks at LLUMC came through. They gave me a packet of information about apartment complexes that offered special rates and two-month furnished rentals to LLUMC patients. They also gave me a stack of hand-outs on things to do while visiting 'The Inland Empire,' as the San Bernardino/Riverside area is known. I was so impressed. These people thought of everything.

I didn't fully understand the meaning of the *Make Man Whole* mission at first. But the more time I spent with the staff, the clearer the meaning became. Loma Linda University Medical Center is a Seventh-day Adventist institution and embraces the Christian philosophy that the human body is the temple of God. Although the senior administrative people at the hospital are members of the Seventh-day Adventist Church, the medical and support staff represent people from all religious backgrounds and beliefs. Yet all seem to embrace the "Make Man Whole" philosophy, which is to restore man to wholeness, physically, emotionally, and spiritually.

At no time during my two-month stay did I feel any pressure to learn more about or participate in any Seventh-day Adventist activities. However, their spiritual presence was felt, and it turned out to be a major factor in my positive experience of LLUMC and in my healing.

I chose to stay at the Redlands Lawn and Tennis Club (RLTC), which was three miles down the road from the hospital. RLTC had beautiful furnished apartments, and the grounds and location were superb. Since my wife Pauline would be joining me, along with other visitors from the east, I felt a comfortable, roomy apartment was important.

How Will We Spend Our Time?

Now that I was committed to spending two months in Southern California away from friends, children, and support systems, I began to wonder how my wife and I would spend our time. I needed to be at the hospital each day, five days a week for my daily treatments; I couldn't wander far off. Would I be terribly bored after the first few days?

LLUMC pays particular attention to patients' physical and emotional needs. All proton treatment patients are automatically enrolled in the new, state-of-the-art, Drayson Physical Fitness Center located on the hospital grounds. This six-acre facility includes four tennis courts, indoor basketball courts and track, two enormous pools, five racquetball courts, and thousands of square feet of physical fitness equipment.

Numerous psychosocial programs have been established to help meet some of the emotional and social needs of patients. I vowed to participate in some of these. After all, I wanted more of the "magic" I experienced at the support group meeting the night before.

Overflowing with information and enriched with new knowledge, I flew home confident, optimistic, and awaiting my start date, October 25, 2000.

CHAPTER 9

My Treatment Begins

He who is outside the door has already got a good part of his journey behind him.

-- Dutch proverb

A Warm California Reception?

My wife and I flew to California on Tuesday, October 24, 2000 to get settled in our new temporary apartment. We landed in Los Angeles, picked up our rental car, and drove east toward Loma Linda. Traffic was horrific, and the 70-mile trip lasted almost three hours. We arrived at Redlands about 9 PM, parked the car, and carried all our gear up to our second floor apartment. Somehow I managed to sprain my back in the process. It was hot – about 85°F – and the air conditioning in our new apartment was broken. Not a great start.

The next morning there was a nasty note on the windshield of my rental car reminding me that I parked in the reserved space of another tenant. How was I to know the spaces were reserved?

We had been there less than 24 hours; we experienced a horrible traffic jam; I sprained my back; our air conditioning didn't work; and I managed to "tick-off" one of my new neighbors. A bad omen?

Treatment Number 1

My first of 38 treatments was on Wednesday, October 25, 2000, at 1:30 PM. My wife, Pauline was invited to observe. This both surprised and delighted me. Despite all my research, I really didn't know what to expect that first day, and neither did my wife.

My instructions were to consume sixteen ounces of water about 20 minutes before the procedure in order to fill my bladder. This actually helps to stretch the bladder and lift it off the prostate and away from the target area of the proton beam (The bladder and prostate are something like a hot air balloon sitting on top of the passenger basket. When the hot air balloon is full of warm air, it lifts and rises off the basket.). I dutifully complied and drank the water.

We were escorted to a changing room where I was told to disrobe and put on a hospital johnny. I could leave my socks on – somehow this comforted me – I don't know why. Pauline joined me in the changing room, to provide company and encouragement. A few minutes later, the door to the changing room opened and the previously treated patient, dressed in his johnny, entered – a slightly awkward moment with Pauline there. It was now time for my first treatment.

Pauline and I walked down the corridor and entered Gantry 3. We were greeted by three Radiation Therapists, Tim, Nick, and Barbara, all beaming with welcoming smiles. I remember thinking, "Sure – it's easy for them to smile – I'm the one having 250 million electron volts shot into my private parts."

I was asked to climb into my pod, which had already been installed on the Gantry treatment table. "How do you know this is my pod?" I asked. They told me my name was written on it and it was bar coded. The bar code was checked by computer in the Gantry room.

Pinching the back of my johnny to hold it closed, lest I show three strangers my best angle, I gingerly climbed into the pod. The smile on the lead therapists face told me that perhaps everybody is modest at first. Later, I would find myself bounding into the pod with an untied johnny flapping in the breeze and my "better side" fully exposed for all to see.

The pod fit perfectly, almost like it was made for me . . . but then, it was.

I was asked to roll over on my left side and was presented with my first "official" balloon – not so bad, but a little embarrassing in front of my wife, especially when they filled it with water from two syringes.

As instructed, I rolled onto my back again and they made an initial adjustment to my position in the pod by tugging on the sheet under me. I was conscious of the water-filled balloon in its "resting place." It felt a little unnatural at first, but not uncomfortable.

Next the pod and platform assembly was slid into the center of the treatment apparatus, and the entire 94-ton gantry began to rotate in order to position the x-ray equipment above me. At first I had the sensation that my pod was rotating and the room was stationary. I found myself hanging on so I wouldn't fall out. I quickly adapted to that phenomenon.

So, there I was 3,000 miles from home, at a hospital in Southern California, lying in my pod, a water balloon in my butt, a sheet covering me, cantilevered into the center of a three-story high, white, cylindrical 94 ton gantry, with two different radiation devices pointed at my pelvic region, about to have billions of protons shot into my prostate. I remember thinking, "What the hell am I doing here?"

At this point Pauline broke down and cried. It seemed to hit her all at once: My diagnosis with prostate cancer; all the research, the phone calls, a two-month move to Southern California; my lying helplessly in this "coffin-like" device, surrounded by hospital technicians dressed in white; and this giant "star wars" machinery rotating around me. She was suddenly struck with thoughts of the mortality of her partner and best friend of 35 years. Death was something we never discussed, or even thought about, because we considered ourselves young, healthy, and physically fit.

With some comforting by the gentle and caring therapists, Pauline regained her composure, and she and the technicians moved behind a radiation barrier. Suddenly there was a short "zap" from the x-ray machine above me. The technicians then pressed a button and the huge gantry rotated ninety degrees. Back behind the barrier and another quick "zap." These low energy x-rays were taken from the top and the side, to find pre-mapped points on my pelvic bones to ensure that I was located in precisely the right spot before the high-energy proton radiation beam was introduced.

While the orthogonal x-rays were being analyzed by the computer, one of the technicians installed three more devices in the gantry machinery that were specifically designed and constructed, or selected for me – the energy modulator, the cerrobend-lead alloy aperture, and the jeweler's wax bolus. These three devices, which help focus the proton beam precisely to the target volume, were bar coded and had to be scanned before the computers would allow the technicians to call for the proton beam.

The size and geometry of these devices were determined from the CT Scan and resulting hologram made of my prostate. The purpose was to ensure that the proton beam was delivered to my prostate, the capsule surrounding my prostate, my seminal vesicles and an extra half-inch margin around the entire package. This is done to tolerances of about plus or minus a half-millimeter. Extraordinary technology!

Based on the information gathered by the two low-energy x-rays, the computer determined the final adjustment that needed to be made to my pod and platform, to place me in the proper position for the proton beam to do its work.

The technicians made this final adjustment and then called in the attending radiation oncologist to check all the settings. The doctor came in, checked the information on the computer screen and the position of the pod in the gantry, and gave his approval to call for the beam. This procedure, including the doctor's final check, would be repeated 37 times.

Next, I heard Tim Holmes, the lead technician, who looked more like a movie star than a radiation therapist, pick up the intercom and tell the accelerator control room, "Gantry 3 is ready for the beam." Tim and his girlfriend, Andrea, would later become good friends.

Tim told me that everything was ready, and that everyone needed to leave the room. "Does that include me?" I quipped. "No," Tim chuckled, "You'll have to stay here."

Now I was alone in the Gantry, and it was totally silent. I remember feeling instantly frightened – and inexplicably sad. Tears began to flow as I lay there helplessly in a custom made pod, with a balloon in my butt, and surrounded by all this machinery. I knew from the orientation tour that the technicians and my wife were in the Gantry 3 control room and were watching me on a TV monitor. I quickly regained my composure so I wouldn't embarrass myself.

Three or four minutes went by and nothing happened. "What do I do now?" I thought. I began to pray. Then I thought about all the research I had done, all the books and articles I had read, the Internet searches, and the interviews. Yes, the interviews! I had spoken with 56 men who had chosen this treatment. "They all can't be wrong," I thought. The more I concentrated on the work I had done that led me to this place, the more I relaxed. I wiped away the tears, smiled and thought, "Thank you, God."

Suddenly the energy modulator wheel began to spin. The whirring sound was eerie, but befitting this "*Star Wars* movie set" I was in. I knew this meant the beam was coming next, and I found myself getting rigid, as if someone were about to punch me in the stomach. But I willed myself to relax. I didn't want to do anything that might move my prostate even an eighth of an inch.

Then I heard the first beep, followed by another, and another . . . about one a second. This was the Geiger counter-type device that confirms the beam is being properly delivered. I remember counting the beeps to estimate the duration of the treatment. It was just about sixty seconds.

The beeping stopped, and the energy modulator whirring slowed and eventually stopped. I felt nothing . . no pain, no discomfort, no burning sensation. It was over. My first treatment was completed. I felt energized; I felt relieved; I was happy; and I knew then I had made the right choice.

Pauline and the Gantry 3 crew came back into the room and congratulated me . . as if I had anything to do with what had just happened.

"OK. Mr. Marckini," Tim said. "Party's over. Time to give us back the balloon. Please roll over on your left side." I complied and he removed the balloon – after draining the water into a small syringe-like reservoir.

I climbed out of the pod, thanked the radiation therapists, and walked back to the dressing room with Pauline. Once there, we hugged, and I said, "We made the right decision."

Each day it was the same routine: Drink the water, climb into the pod, receive my balloon, and get zapped. Nothing to it! I was into the routine, and it was a piece of cake.

Early Treatment Time

I quickly learned that being treated in the middle of the day was undesirable. It didn't allow me to schedule golf, or for us to go sightseeing in the beautiful Inland Empire. So, I asked the manager of the Proton Treatment Unit if it was possible to shift to an earlier time slot. He suggested that I take it up with the radiation therapists in Gantry 3. I did as he suggested, and a few days later, I had a 7:20 AM time slot. This was perfect, because it gave us the entire day to have fun. It also gave us a three-day weekend, and plenty of time to explore a large part of Southern California.

I didn't know how lucky I was to get this early time slot until later, when I learned that, as the day progressed, the probability of the schedule becoming disrupted by late arrivals, equipment problems, and computer glitches increased dramatically.

Golf, Guitar, and Grazing

The early time slot allowed me to complete treatment before breakfast and then have the rest of the day to exercise and play.

I learned there are about 30 golf courses within short driving distance of Loma Linda. The Redlands Country Club, one of the oldest golf courses in Southern California, was about five minutes from our apartment. This private club offers LLUMC outpatients temporary memberships at a reasonable price. So, it looked like my golf needs would be taken care of.

Next I searched for and found a music store and guitar teacher to help me improve my skills with that uncompromising six stringed instrument.

The Redlands, California Chamber of Commerce and the local AAA were most helpful in providing us with information about local tourist attractions, maps, and driving directions.

There are lots of excellent restaurants in the area including Citrone, Greensleaves, Mario's Place, Seville, The Mission Inn, Napoli, Clara's, The Claim Jumper, and Mimi's. Pauline and I set out to visit each one of them. We never had to travel any further than San

Bernardino, Redlands, or Riverside for superb dining that would satisfy the taste of even the most discriminating gourmet.

My Routine

For the next two months I arose at 6:30 AM, showered, drank my 24 ounces of water (16 ounces were required, but I wanted a little insurance), had my treatment, and was back at the apartment in time to make coffee and awaken my wife to plan the day . . hardly the scenario one would expect for treating a life-threatening disease.

Each patient is encouraged to meet with his radiation oncologist weekly. I met with Dr. Rossi on Wednesdays, but since the treatment was going so smoothly, I rarely had anything of consequence to talk about. I was fascinated by proton treatment, so I used the meetings as opportunities to learn as much as I could about proton treatment technology.

Dr. Rossi is unique as a physician. He is as humble as he is brilliant. He has the ability to put you at ease with his words and his demeanor. No question is too difficult, or too stupid. I liked him the first day I met him at the initial consult, and my admiration for him grew with each meeting.

Pauline joined me for many of the meetings, and her questions were answered as well. I actually found myself looking forward my weekly meetings with Dr. Rossi. It almost felt like I was spending quality time with an old friend.

Sharon Hoyle was my Nurse/Case Manager. I first met her by phone when I was doing my research. She could not have been more helpful to me. Sharon is the model of what every nurse should strive to be. If Florence Nightingale could be reincarnated, she would come back as Sharon Hoyle.

Somewhere in my travels I came across something called "The Florence Nightingale Pledge."

I solemnly pledge myself before God and presence of this assembly: To pass my life in purity and to practice my profession faithfully. I will abstain from whatever is deleterious and mischievous and will not take or knowingly administer any harmful drug. I will do all in my power to maintain and elevate the standard of my profession and will hold in confidence all personal matters committed to my keeping and family affairs coming to my knowledge in the practice of my calling. With loyalty will I endeavor to aid the physician in his work, and devote myself to the welfare of those committed to my care.

This describes Sharon Hoyle perfectly, and influenced me to give her the nickname "Flo," which I use in my correspondence with her to this day.

The Nutritionist

During the first week of treatment, patients are asked to meet with the Department of Radiation Medicine Nutritionist. While it is not essential to change your diet during treatment, avoiding certain foods could help prevent some temporary, minor intestinal problems, such as diarrhea.

Pauline and I met with Stella, a wonderful Jamaican lady with a smile that won us over before she spoke a word. Soft gospel music was playing on her portable stereo, and I had a good feeling about the meeting we were about to have.

We learned that Stella was a Seventh-day Adventist, and as such, she followed the Adventist diet regimen, which is largely vegetarian, with other restrictions such as no caffeine or alcohol. Thankfully, she didn't tell me I had to temporarily curtail my meat, caffeine and wine intake during treatment. Eliminating meat I could possibly handle, but giving up breathing would be easier than skipping my morning coffee ritual and my evening glass of wine with dinner.

Stella gave me some information on a healthy diet for life, with some specific suggestions for minor diet changes during treatment, including avoiding such foods as nuts and prunes, and green leafy vegetables.

I can't say that I strictly followed Stella's recommendations. During treatment I ate much what I usually ate, and had no problems. I did hear of a couple of patients who experienced some problems with diarrhea as a result of *not* following Stella's suggestions.

Our diet is generally healthy. We rarely eat red meat, eggs, or butter. Chicken, turkey, and fish are regular staples. Salads, fresh vegetables, and bean soups are also a part of our regular diet.

Breakfast typically consists of a banana, orange juice, oat, bran or wheat cereals with skim milk, and of course . . . coffee. A man needs a few vices in his life!

I later learned that many proton patients have life-changing experiences at Loma Linda that go beyond being cured of cancer. Often this begins with Stella's tips on diet and nutrition, and her explanation of how important this is to our general health and longevity. Most patients, I learned, complete their treatment at Loma Linda leaving with a commitment to a healthier overall lifestyle. We were no exception.

Emotional Fitness

Psychological or emotional health has been shown to both enhance physical health and strengthen the immune system, which helps prevent disease and hasten the healing process.

As mentioned earlier, *radiation works by damaging the cancer cells' DNA, preventing the cells from reproducing. Healthy cells damaged by radiation typically repair themselves and reproduce, while the damaged cancer cells eventually die off. Clearly both of these processes – healthy cell repair and cancer cell death – are enhanced by a healthy emotional state and a positive mental attitude.* Scientific studies have shown that emotional and psychological factors can positively or negatively impact the immune system's ability to fend-off diseases of all kinds, including cancer.

LLUMC has established a Social Work Department within Radiation Medicine as part of their effort to provide emotional/psychological support to patients while in treatment – clearly an integral part of their mission "To Make Man Whole."

The entire atmosphere at Loma Linda is consistent with their mission, and the personal support patients feel while in treatment goes far beyond the social work department. It is present everywhere – in the medical staff, reception, billing, insurance, and even the cafeteria.

I have often been critical of the over-dependency of our population on psychologists and psychotherapists, and the small percentage of practitioners who actually do their patients any good (I have seen some people severely harmed by their psychotherapists). However, I *do* believe there is a place for competent psychologists, psychiatrists and social workers in our society.

The psychosocial programs at LLUMC are leading edge, and they are amazingly effective. At the heart of these programs is the Wednesday night support group meeting.

When I was doing my research and interviewing proton patients, the Wednesday night support group meetings were frequently mentioned. I heard, "You must attend," or, "Don't miss a single one." I put that advice aside, because of my belief, "real men don't do support groups." I had visions of fifty people sitting in a circle, holding hands and singing Kumbaya. I couldn't have been more wrong. My experience while there for my consult convinced me of that.

Since my treatments started on a Wednesday, I had the opportunity to attend my second Wednesday night support group meeting – the first for Pauline. We arrived just after 5:30, and at Pauline's suggestion, planned to stay for an hour and then go out to dinner. We helped ourselves to some refreshments and entered the room. Once again, it was packed with about 90 people sitting around rectangular tables, and a few sitting in folding chairs randomly placed in any available space. There were no empty chairs, and others were standing, so we decided to stand near the door so we could make our quiet exit.

The mood in the room was festive. People were laughing; and that didn't make sense to Pauline, even though I had explained to her my experience of this meeting two weeks before.

Gerry Troy stood up and introduced himself. With a calm and sincere voice, he welcomed all of us, reminded us to help ourselves to some refreshments, and told us the location of the rest rooms. The latter, I learned is important, as urinary urgency is a common temporary side effect of *any* radiation delivered to the prostate bed.

Gerry then made some announcements about group activities. Next, he read a poem and a couple of jokes, all sent to him by former patients, expressly for this meeting. These were well received, and we found ourselves laughing with the rest of the group.

He then asked if there were any Graduates in the audience. About seven hands went up. He called on one of them – a gentleman about 60 years old from Arizona named Richard – who stood up and told his story. Richard began by announcing his pretreatment PSA and Gleason score. Then he talked about how his prostate cancer was discovered; his shock and disbelief; the meeting with his urologist who recommended surgery; his investigation of the alternatives; his discovery of proton treatment; the help he received from former proton patients; his physician's unprofessional behavior when he heard Richard had chosen proton treatment ("Find yourself another urologist when you return!"); his wonderful experience of both treatment and his two month stay in southern California. He then reported his most recent PSA, 0.9, which drew spontaneous applause from the audience.

This process was repeated six more times. The PSAs, Gleason Scores, and home states varied, but the stories were similar. They all looked beyond their urologist's first recommendation, did their homework, investigated the options, got help from former proton patients, and had a positive experience at Loma Linda.

Gerry then asked if there were any visitors who were not patients. Surprisingly, four hands went up. One at a time people stood up to tell their story. They had been recently diagnosed with prostate cancer and were investigating their options. Two were from California and two from out of state. They were there for consults with radiation oncologists and to see first hand what proton treatment was all about. Each stood, reported his numbers, and talked about where they were in their decision making process. Each was there with his wife, or significant other, which was the case for most of the other men in the room. Thank God for this support from our wives.

Next Gerry asked if there were any Newbies present. I raised my hand, along with about twelve other men. One at a time we stood up and told our story. We ranged in age from early 50s to late 70s and hailed from several U.S. States – one was from Canada. One of the twelve had been fitted for his pod, but had not begun treatment. The rest of us were in the early stages of our treatment. I found myself comfortably talking to this group of "brothers," and I drew a few chuckles when I told them about the 56 interviews.

Others who were in treatment raised their hands and offered comments, observations, poems, and songs they had written about their experience of the pod and the rectal balloon. These two subjects seemed to receive a lot of attention, always in a humorous vein.

I noticed one young woman sitting in the room, and one side of her face appeared to be sunburned. I learned that she was being treated at the Proton Treatment Center for an inoperable tumor on the optic nerve of her left eye. Others in the room were there for tumors on the brain or eye. And one was being treated for macular degeneration. Most who raised their hands and spoke that night were prostate cancer patients. I later learned that prostate cancer patients represent about 65% of those treated at the Loma Linda Proton Treatment Center.

A guest speaker made a presentation that evening. It was Dr. Dan Miller, chief physicist at the Medical Center. He used overhead slides and a white board to explain in great detail how protons are generated; how they are intentionally "spilled" from the accelerator and directed to the treatment rooms; how the narrow beam is expanded; and how the customized devices shape the beam precisely to each patient's targeted area. Dr. Miller had invited questions at the beginning of his presentation, and the crowd was not bashful. He answered dozens of questions during his talk and for about 20 minutes after it ended.

I looked at my watch and discovered it was 8:30 PM. We had been there for 3 hours and it seemed like 15 minutes! "If all the Wednesday night support group meetings are like this one," I thought to myself, "I'm not going to miss one of them." They were – and I didn't.

My experience of the leading edge psychosocial programs at LLUMC, such as the Wednesday night support group was a major factor in a life-changing decision I later made to form a support group that would become international in scope, and impact the lives of thousands of people.

Today, well over a hundred patients in treatment attend the weekly support group meetings at the Proton Treatment Center. And, just as in the past, it is standing room only, every Wednesday night.

Gerry Troy has since moved on to the University of Florida Proton Therapy Institute. He is realizing his dream of taking the programs he helped pioneer at Loma Linda and bringing them to other medical institutions. In collaboration with Loma Linda and Shands, Gerry intends to share this program with other proton treatment facilities as they are established in the U.S. and abroad.

Physical Fitness

LLUMC's mission "To Make Man Whole" is evident in every aspect of the patient's experience during treatment. They teach patients that staying physically fit greatly benefits the immune system and aids the healing process. A strong immune system also helps prevent a cancer recurrence.

When I sat through the orientation session during my first visit, I was given a large packet of information on a wide range of subjects including places to stay in the community during treatment, points of interest, technical papers on proton treatment, maps of the area and other general information. I was reminded that, in California, at 57 years of age, I had already been a "senior citizen" for two years. Not a pleasant thought for me, as I considered myself "approaching middle age." Nevertheless, there were benefits to being a senior at Loma Linda. Among them were discounts at the hospital cafeteria and preferred parking spaces at the Medical Center.

Another part of the packet of information I received was a certificate that authorized my wife and me to use the expansive, state-of-the-art physical fitness facility on the hospital grounds called the Drayson Center. This complex is named in honor of Dr. Ronald and Grace Drayson, who provided the lead gift that was used to help build the fitness center.

The $16 million complex is a modern, 100,000 square-foot facility serving students, faculty, and patients. The Drayson Center's mission is to provide opportunities for enhancement of the quality of life within this community through a wide variety of social, recreational, and health-building activities, all consistent with LLUMC's mission, "To Make Man Whole."

Pauline and I were already in reasonably good physical condition. We both exercised regularly, and followed a generally healthy lifestyle.

We were encouraged to visit the Drayson Center and take advantage of all it had to offer while I was there for treatment – and we did.

Each day we would visit the center and spend about 90 minutes working out. We began our workout by spending a half hour on one of the treadmills. Then we switched to the fitness equipment to do upper and lower body exercises.

We found ourselves looking forward to our daily routine at the Drayson Center, and during our eight-week stay, we increased both our physical strength and our endurance.

Following our late morning workout, we fell into another routine: Eating lunch at the hospital cafeteria.   Seventh-day

Adventists take a healthy diet very seriously, and that naturally extends to the hospital cafeteria.

Hospital food has historically been considered bland and unpalatable. Not so at Loma Linda. The food at the LLUMC cafeteria was outstanding – fresh salads, fresh fruits, fresh vegetables, home made soups, cooked meals of all sorts and a wide variety of beverages; but no meat and no caffeine. This last part was a little hard getting used to, as coffee and a diet coke had been a regular part of our daily routine for years.

'Stealth' Health

Without realizing it, I had been gently led down three very important paths of LLUMC's approach to treating the whole person. Within the first few days of my stay, I was eating a healthier diet, exercising daily, and participating in programs aimed at nurturing my emotional well-being.

When I returned home in December 2000, I was stronger, healthier, and more physically fit. And, as it turned out, I had a new perspective on spirituality and my faith.

Little wonder that proton patients go through "withdrawal" as they near the end of their treatment.

The Spiritual Side

I have mentioned that LLUMC is a Seventh-day Adventist institution. Yet, except for the cross on the tower over the main entrance, some statues on the medical center and university grounds, and some paintings in the lobby depicting Jesus Christ healing the sick, there are few outward signs of the religious side of this institution. True, senior administrative staff at the hospital and university are Adventists, and things tended to quiet down considerably on Saturday, the Adventists' Sabbath, but there was no evidence of anyone 'advertising' or 'pushing' the Seventh-day Adventist faith, either overtly or covertly. Yet, there was clearly a spiritual atmosphere permeating this institution.

The dictionary defines spiritual as "sacred, devotional or ecclesiastical, not lay or temporal," and that aptly describes the Loma

Linda environment my wife and I experienced during those eight weeks.

Pauline at that time was Protestant, and I was Catholic. We attended Catholic Mass while at Loma Linda. And, during our stay, we found our faith taking on new meaning and a new importance in our lives. Perhaps some of this was related to our coming face to face with my mortality. But there was also a component heavily influenced by the spiritual side of Loma Linda.

It is clearly there, though I cannot put proper words on paper to describe it. All patients experience it. It shows up in the way we are treated by the staff – doctors, nurses, administrative people, security personnel, and even parking lot attendants. It is in the cafeteria when a table of eight members of the medical staff, bow their heads and offer a silent prayer of thanks before a meal. It is evident at the Wednesday night support group meetings. It is even present at the Drayson Center where people go to strengthen their bodies.

Since my treatment ended in December 2000, I have had the opportunity to communicate with thousands of current and former LLUMC patients. A surprising number of them talk openly about how "God sent me to Loma Linda." Or, it was "Divine intervention," or "Divine guidance" that led them to Loma Linda. Most – Christians and non-Christians alike – have had some kind of spiritual awakening as a result of their experience at LLUMC.

One patient I met there is a good example. When his treatment ended he found himself much more "connected" with his Jewish faith and with God. He changed his lifestyle dramatically following treatment; improved his eating habits and became more physically fit; sold his large home and refocused his life on helping others through philanthropic activities. Today, he is a much happier person as a result of this "transformation" that began at Loma Linda.

Dr. J. Lynn Martell, Vice President of Advancement at Loma Linda, would attend the Wednesday night meetings whenever he was in town. That's where I met him. We would later become close friends. Lynn loved to meet the patients and help keep the Wednesday meeting upbeat. He regularly spoke to the group, welcoming Newbies and congratulating Graduates and Alumni. He would often tell us, "We are a religious institution and we make no apologies for that. And, you are not here by accident."

Dr. Martell was absolutely right. Along with most of the others, I felt I was meant to be there. A Higher Power clearly led me to Loma Linda and to an experience that has had a profound impact on my life, a life that would never be the same again.

"Lover's Groan" and Other Short Term Side Effects

During the first few weeks of treatment my wife and I continued our normal sexual relationship as we were told we could. Around week six however, I began to notice a burning sensation deep in my groin, during orgasm. This became increasingly more unpleasant as my treatments progressed.

Dr. Rossi explained that my prostate was being irradiated every day by the powerful proton beam, that the discomfort I was experiencing was normal, and that it would dissipate after treatment ended.

When I compared notes with other men in treatment, I learned that many had similar experiences. One jokingly referred to this unique experience as "lover's groan," and the term seemed to stick. As Dr. Rossi predicted, the discomfort disappeared a few weeks after treatment ended.

About the same time the "lover's groan" appeared, I began to experience some slight urinary burning and increased urgency to urinate. At night I found myself having to make three or four bathroom trips. During the day it was worse. At times I couldn't go much more than a half hour without having to visit the rest room.

That wasn't so bad, but things got a little more complicated when I was playing golf one day about seven weeks into treatment. I went to the golf course by myself that day and was matched up with three women. There were only two restrooms on the course, and I knew I was going to get into trouble as the urinary urgency was just about at its peak, with relief stops needed about every 20 minutes.

At first I managed by lagging behind, between holes, and sneaking into the bushes as the other three walked ahead. As the match progressed and we made friends, the three of them began to wait for me out of courtesy, denying me my much-needed relief.

I am a high handicap golfer, so I often hit my fair share of balls to landing areas other than the fairway. But never had I intentionally directed balls into the woods . . . until that day. At least once on every hole I would wind up and crack one deep into the brush or over a hill behind a sand trap, and then gingerly trot after it to get my blessed relief.

My golf partners must have thought it a bit odd when I frequently lined up about 45 degrees from the direction of the green and swatted one deep into the woods. I suspect they talk about that 'crazy guy' to this day.

Things were a little easier off the golf course, but I *did* realize that Loma Linda prostate cancer radiation patients all have one thing in common. We know exactly where every public rest room is located in San Bernardino County. You can be driving down Orange Street, feel the urge and be in the rest room of the small eclectic sandwich shop in minutes. On Redlands Boulevard I charted six easy rest stops on the three-mile run between my apartment and the hospital. At a support group meeting, one of the patients produced a map of the community with every public restroom identified within a five square mile radius of the hospital. The audience laughed loudly; then several attendees requested a copy.

My problem with urinary urgency and slight burning was short lived. Dr. Rossi prescribed Pyridium Plus, which took care of the problem until it disappeared on its own about four weeks after treatment ended. This particular medication has an interesting side effect – it turns your urine bright orange. Not a problem unless you are in a public restroom and someone catches sight of your fluorescent discharge. This earned me a few strange looks.

CHAPTER 10

The Fun Part of Spending Eight Weeks in Southern California

"A truly happy person is one who can enjoy the scenery on a detour."

-- Unknown

Getting Into the Swing of Things

Loma Linda provides a list of dozens of furnished rooms and apartments to stay in during treatment. As mentioned earlier, Pauline and I chose the Redlands Lawn and Tennis Club, a condo/apartment facility, three miles down the road from the hospital with tennis courts, swimming pool, and exercise room in a beautifully landscaped, gated community.

We enjoyed the 'freedom' of apartment living for eight weeks and made friends with two of our neighbors. These friendships continue to this day. One couple was a young man who was a civilian employee of the Department of Defense and his wife Rene, a German National who was learning to speak English. They were lots of fun. Her mistakes with the English language provided much of the entertainment while we were together.

It took me quite a while, for example, to understand the word "reeseep," which she used several times in a conversation one day. Finally, I had to ask her, "Rene, what is this word, 'reeseep?'" She said indignantly, "Reeseep, spelled r-e-c-i-p-e, reeseep!" There were many more of these gems in her vocabulary.

119

Rene also picked up some slang and some colloquialisms along the way. One was the term "gang bang." She thought it meant, "a confusing situation." After having a pipe break in her apartment one day, the landlord sent a plumber, a carpenter, and a clean up crew to help fix things. At dinner that night she told us, "You should have seen it, the plumber, the carpenter, and the clean up guys. We had a real gang bang in my apartment today."

Pauline spent much of her time reading, walking, and learning to knit. The latter provided me with much amusement, as she chose a complex pattern for her first project and managed to disassemble it and start over about thirty times during our stay, effectively 'wearing out' the yarn.

The Drayson center occupied most of our mornings. Golf, guitar lessons, sight seeing, reading, tennis, and other activities filled the afternoons.   Evenings were often spent exploring the many wonderful restaurants in the Inland Empire.

Golf

A golf practice range was located roughly midway between our apartment and the hospital a mile down the road. The first week of our stay, I loaded my clubs into the rental car, drove there and introduced myself to the teaching pro, Jim Becker, who managed the facility. I told him I was going to be in town for a couple of months and was interested in some lessons. His response was, "Let me guess, you have prostate cancer and you're being treated with protons over at Loma Linda." I was dumbfounded, and asked how he knew. He told me he's had a couple hundred golf students come through over the past few years, mostly men in their 50s to their 80s, and all with the same story. Jim and I became friends during our stay, and the five lessons I paid for somehow stretched to twelve – at no extra cost. He also provided me with introductions to the pros at several local golf clubs, including two new PGA courses. I played all of them at substantially discounted greens fees, thanks to Jim's influence.

Travel, Tours, Restaurants and More

Pauline and I visited San Diego on one of our three-day weekends. Pauline fell in love with the giant pandas at the San Diego Zoo. I was fascinated by the killer whales on our visit to Sea World.

Our friends Bob and Barbara Destino live in Mission Viejo, which is about an hour southwest of Loma Linda – with no traffic (All commuting times in southern California should be multiplied by two or three for rush hour traffic).

Pauline grew up in northern Vermont with Barbara, and they have always been close friends. Her husband Bob and I have also become friends over the years. We spent an enjoyable three-day weekend playing golf, attending church with them, reminiscing, and catching up on the events of our lives. It was a truly enjoyable weekend. I had to keep reminding myself that I was there having treatment for a life-threatening disease.

One Sunday morning after church, we decided to visit one of the local attractions listed in the sightseeing pamphlets provided by the LLUMC Social Work Group. The Morey Mansion was only a few blocks from our apartment in Redlands. When we pulled up we saw only one car in the parking area, suggesting to us that perhaps it was closed on Sunday. We pulled in anyway.

No one answered the front door bell, so we walked around back and were greeted by a lady working in a beautiful garden. I presumed she was one of the groundskeepers, and asked if the mansion was open for tours on Sunday. She smiled and told us the mansion hadn't been open for tours for three years. She and her husband purchased the mansion, and they had spent the last three years restoring it.

I was embarrassed; I apologized for the intrusion and explained how the whole thing happened. To our surprise, she asked if we would like to see her home now that it had been fully restored. We answered, "Of course!" And then the most amazing thing happened: She suggested we begin on the top floor and work our way down, and, as soon as she was finished in the yard, she would join us.

At first we felt uncomfortable walking through the private home of a perfect stranger. The home was extraordinary – fully restored in every detail. The lady joined us, and spent an hour sharing the history of the mansion and the restoration details. To this day, we look back on that event and try to picture something similar happening anyplace else on the planet. And we both came to the same conclusion – it could never happen.

The restaurants were superb in the Redlands, San Bernardino, and Riverside areas. We never had time during those eight weeks to visit all of them, but on each return visit, we manage to add more to our list.

In early December we took a ride on the brand new rotating tramway gondola, which brought us to the top of Mount San Jacinto near Palm Springs. San Jacinto is the second tallest mountain in southern California with an elevation of 10,804 feet at the peak. This is definitely not a ride for those with "weak knees," like me, but the spectacular view of the Palm Springs area is worth it.

One of the highlights of our stay was a visit to the Crystal Cathedral in Garden Grove, California. It was a Sunday morning service with Dr. Robert Schuller. For years we had watched Dr. Schuller on TV. It was a special treat to be there in the front row, hearing him preach, and listening to the Crystal Cathedral organ and choir.

Tenth Anniversary Celebration

We were fortunate to have been at Loma Linda in November of 2000. This was the tenth anniversary of the opening of the Proton Treatment Center. The celebration was held on November 12, and it lasted all day. There were tours of the facility, chamber music, a luncheon, and a reception hosted by Dr. Lyn Behrens, Chief Executive Officer of Loma Linda University Adventist Health Science Center, the parent organization for the Medical Center and University. Also hosting the event were Dr. James Slater, the Pioneer of proton therapy, and Dr. Jerry Slater, Chairman of the Department of Radiation.

Later in the day there were presentations given by the above people, welcoming the large gathering of current and former patients of the Proton Treatment Center as well as faculty, hospital staff, and other guests. Speakers reviewed the history of the project, the challenges, the successes over the past ten years, and plans for the future. I learned that the tiny proton particle is one of the most powerful forces of nature for curing diseases of all types, and that research is underway at Loma Linda to unleash that power . . . the only obstacle being adequate funding for proton research.

Congressman Jerry Lewis, a key sponsor of the original facility was unable to attend, but spoke to us by videotape from his Washington office.

The chief physicist on the project from the FermiLab, Phil Livdahl, also spoke. A humble man, he described the technical challenges and his partnership with Dr. James Slater. He told us that ironically, shortly after the project was completed, he was diagnosed with prostate cancer and became the first prostate cancer patient treated with protons at the new facility. Ten years later he was still cancer free. Years later, I would become friends with this great man.

One young woman, Jennifer Gardner, told the story of how she was diagnosed, at age 17, with an inoperable brain tumor. She and her family were told there was no hope and that she would die. Her aunt, a nurse at Loma Linda, persuaded her to talk with the doctors there about proton treatment. She did, and four years later, as she told her story, she was cancer free, and studying to become a radiation oncologist; there wasn't a dry eye in that packed auditorium.

An organic chemistry professor, Dr. Roy Butler spoke of his experience with proton treatment for his prostate cancer; how he managed to teach his class at Norwich University 3,000 miles away while being treated; and how he arranged a sabbatical to teach at Redlands University and remain in the Loma Linda area for an additional year. Dr. Butler recounted the humorous side of his treatment and he quickly had the audience laughing.

During his sabbatical, while teaching at Redlands University, Roy spent considerable time at LLUMC, absorbing everything he could about the technology of proton therapy. Using this information, he produced a comprehensive document, explaining the technology in layman's terms. He titled his work, *The Patient Proton*. This important document would later appear on my website, www.protonbob.com.

At the end of the program, the MC asked all those in the audience who had been helped by proton treatment to come up to the stage. About 200 of us gathered there. A singer walked up to the microphone and in a booming, baritone voice sang *You'll Never Walk Alone*. As I stood there on stage with the others, the tears began to flow. I was not alone. Two hundred of us, mostly men and mostly former prostate cancer patients were standing there with tears of hope in our eyes. And most of our family members, along with the faculty and staff in the audience had their handkerchiefs out too. It was a powerfully emotional experience.

At the conclusion of the program, Dr. J. Lynn Martell walked to the podium and offered a prayer of thanksgiving. During that prayer I remember thinking, Pauline and I should plan to be here for the 15th and 20th anniversaries. How's that for optimism?

Thanksgiving Break and Friends Visit

Halfway through treatment Pauline and I flew home for the long Thanksgiving weekend. Our friends were a little surprised to see me so rested and tanned. I think they expected me to be pale, skinny and bald. On Saturday evening they held a surprise party for me, where they presented me with a bouquet – of balloons. This "arrangement" consisted of 20 deflated balloons, representing the number of treatments completed, and 18 inflated balloons for the number of treatments remaining. I remember thinking, "What great friends we have!"

My wife stayed home the next two weeks at my request, to make room for several of my friends. Steve Kane, Frank Esposito, Joe Bruno, Paul Souza, and Ed Urquhart flew to California to keep me company during my "ordeal."

My buddy Steve Kane, from Philadelphia, came first. He's a former high school basketball coach and physical fitness "nut." He thought he had "died and gone to heaven" when I brought him to the Drayson Fitness Center.

Steve and I are on opposite sides of the political spectrum and at that time the presidential election of 2000 was still in contention, as the ballots were being recounted in Florida for the second or third time. We had many heated discussions during his visit, and we are still good friends.

Following Steve's visit, my four friends from the east coast arrived. They brought their golf clubs, and we have photographs and memories of their visit that will last a lifetime.

While they were at Loma Linda, I arranged for them to tour the Proton Treatment unit, and to observe one of my 7:20AM treatments. After the tour, all five of us crowded into the changing room where I slipped into my hospital johnny. Then they accompanied me into the Gantry where I climbed into my pod to prepare for my daily dose of protons. All the while, my friend Ed was snapping photos with his digital camera. Here I prepared a little surprise for them.

My friend Joe Bruno and I have played practical jokes on each other over the years. It was Joe who arranged for the unique balloon bouquet. Prior to my friends' visit, I had rehearsed some dialogue with Tim Holmes, the lead radiation therapist who would be inserting my rectal balloon that morning.

All four of my friends were huddled together on one side of the gantry while the three therapists were going about their business. Tim asked me to roll over on my left side, in order to allow him to insert the infamous balloon. Just as he began the process, I leaned over my right shoulder and asked, "Tim, all the time you've been shoving the balloon up there, I never asked. What do you call this procedure?" He replied, "Mr. Marckini, we call this the *Bruno* procedure." That caught my friends completely by surprise, and certainly lightened things up. I was later told that the laughter could be heard in the Level B waiting room a good distance away.

Weekly Note to Friends

Another way I occupied my time during those eight weeks was by writing weekly status reports to friends on my computer and distributing them by e-mail. I shared not only the status of my treatment regimen and the things Pauline and I were doing to occupy our time, but also some of my observations of living in southern California.

I tried to find the humor in what was happening to me and around me, and share it in my reports. My friends were entertained by these notes and they were sharing them with others. Each week I was asked to add more e-mail addresses to my distribution list. By the time I completed treatment, I was sending copies of my weekly notes to seventy-five people. Here is an excerpt from one report where I was making some observations of life in Southern California

"Driving down the highway the other day, I noticed a sign. It said: 'Fine for illegally driving in the carpool lane: $271.' Now

try to stretch your imagination. Why . . . how . . . under what conditions could any rational human being or governmental agency choose a fine of $271 for driving in a carpool lane? Why not $300, or $250, or even $275? But $271?? Only in California!

Did you know that there were 261 earthquakes in California last week? This is a fact, check out this website: http://quake.wr.usgs.gov/recenteqs/. Most of these are only detectable by seismic equipment, but the fact remains – this place is movin' and shakin'. I knew California had more quakes than most other states, but I had no idea there were that many. Why would anybody want to live here?

We saw a nice Christmas touch around the corner from our apartment this week . . . a Christmas tree on a front lawn decorated entirely with Budweiser Beer cans. Only in California.

One of the popular radio shows out here is the Phil Henry Show. He invites controversial characters to call in, and then for other callers to challenge them. Last Tuesday a car dealer from Beverly Hills called to complain about the Stage 2 power alert in California. He was upset that he had to turn off the power to his Christmas Manger scene at his dealership. Seems that he had the infant in the manger outfitted with a mechanical arm that handed out free drink certificates for a local bar. They really know how to celebrate the spirit of Christmas out here in California.

Another guy called in and told Phil that he was suing his wife because she made him buy leather pants to wear to an outdoor rock concert. They were sitting on metal folding chairs, the pants ripped in the seat, and he apparently froze his private parts. He claims this has interfered with his ability to have a connubial relationship with his wife and is suing her for lack of consortium. Only in California.

And how about the weird names Southern Californians give to their cities . . . Temecula, La Jolla, Topanga, Alhambra, Chula Vista, Coalinga, and Rancho Cucamonga . What ever happened to real 'nuts-and-bolts' American city names like Flint, Bayonne, and Malden? I'm telling you, they're nuts out here."

Christmas in Loma Linda

Near the end of my treatment, we were approaching the Christmas holidays. I will never forget what happened at a Wednesday night support group meeting in mid December. Dr. Martell, who attended most of the meetings stood up and asked the group of a hundred or so, "How many of you, will still be here during the Christmas Holidays?" A bunch of hands went up. Next, he said, "No one should spend Christmas in a lonely apartment. I'd like to invite you all to come to my home and have Christmas dinner with me and my family."

I was flabbergasted. It felt like a scene from "It's a Wonderful Life." I tried to imagine a senior administrative official at Johns Hopkins or the Mayo Clinic inviting dozens of patients to his home for Christmas Dinner.

About 65 people accepted Lynn's invitation and spent Christmas with the Martell family. I didn't learn until later that Lynn's invitation that night was spontaneous. He hadn't discussed it with his wife. I could not imagine telling my wife, "Oh honey, I just invited 65 strangers to spend Christmas day with us. What will you be serving for dinner?"

Dr. Martell and his lovely wife Karen have continued this tradition. Last Christmas they entertained 86 patients and their families in their home. Tables were set up in every room in the house including bedrooms and a bathroom. All had a great meal and a good time. Yes, even in the 21st century it can be 'A Wonderful Life.'

Let's Form a Support Group

During treatment at Loma Linda, I became friends with several men who were also receiving treatment. This included Bill Day, a recently retired Northwest Airlines pilot from Washington state; Roy Butler, the brilliant chemistry professor from Vermont who became a 'proton groupie;' Dan Anderson, a magazine publisher from Chicago; Jerry Klein, a scientist and professional photographer from Washington state; Cal Jones, Deputy District Attorney for San Bernardino County; Bill Hansell, County Commissioner for Umatilla County Oregon, and many more.

As we approached the end of our eight-week treatment period, we talked about ways to keep in touch, to maintain our friendships, and to communicate about side effects, post-treatment PSAs and other factors involving our recovery. I recommended that we form an e-mail support group. No one else would have to know. After all, 'real men' don't join support groups. This would be our own little secret club, like in the Robin Williams movie, *Dead Poet's Society*.

Little did we know at the time, that this little venture was about to take on a life of its own.

CHAPTER 11

Life After Proton Treatment

Only those who will risk going too far can possibly find out how far one can go.

-- T.S. Eliot

As I write this chapter it is six years since I received proton treatment. If one were to ask me if my life has changed as a result of my treatment for prostate cancer, I would say, "Are you kidding? The answer is *yes*, and all for the better!"

Side Effects

As far as side effects are concerned, I can truly say they have been minimal and temporary. The short-term urinary urgency and slight burning during urination left me within a few weeks after treatment ended. Bladder control is normal. There has been one positive benefit of my treatment – my prostate has shrunk in size from the proton radiation. I find I no longer get up at night to visit the bathroom. And thankfully, our sex life is as good as it was before treatment.

When the prostate is removed during surgery, there is no more ejaculate during orgasm for those who are fortunate enough to remain potent. Similarly, when the prostate is bombarded with radiation, it is common for the volume of ejaculate to be significantly reduced, often to zero. Most of us do not see this as a problem. And some see it as a distinct advantage!

The radiation "tan mark" entry point on each of my hips roughly conformed to the profile of the lead alloy aperture used to shape the beam during treatment. I never experienced any sunburn pain or discomfort from these marks, and they disappeared after a few months.

About a year after treatment ended, I experienced some rectal bleeding. I noticed it following a bowel movement. There was about a thimble-full of blood in the bowl. I had been told during treatment that this could happen and that it was quite normal.

I spoke with my doctor at LLUMC and he explained to me that the anterior (inside) wall of the rectum can be in the "line of fire" of the proton beam, if it is within the 12 millimeter (half inch) margin around the prostate that is targeted during treatment. The balloon, which inflates the rectum, protects the rest of the circumference of the rectum from seeing any radiation damage.

As this healthy tissue repairs itself, there is a phenomenon called radiation-induced neovascularization. New blood vessels form in the rectal wall, and periodically some blood vessels near the surface leak blood, or a scab will "slough off." This condition is not uncommon, it is self-limiting, and it almost always goes away after a few months. I noticed some blood in my stool about once a month for 18 months, as the condition gradually diminished and disappeared. For the past four years there has been no blood.

Occasionally, I'm told, the bleeding can become a nuisance and may require a painless out-patient procedure called argon plasma coagulation, sometimes referred to as "APC." Rarely does this condition require more than that.

Post Treatment PSA Trend

Four months after treatment ended, I scheduled a blood test and DRE (digital rectal exam) as directed. The DRE was normal. In fact my urologist, who was a proton skeptic before I was treated, told me my prostate felt as soft and supple as a much younger man's. "I assume that's good?" I asked. "Of course," was his answer. He told me my prostate had actually shrunk and that it felt normal and healthy. Good news!

Waiting for that first PSA was torture. I remember calling my urologist to learn the results. Lots of things were going through my mind. What if it didn't work? What if my PSA is still rising beyond the 8.0 pretreatment level? I never felt any pain or discomfort during treatment – maybe the beam wasn't working and I didn't know it. Maybe this proton thing is a big scam – after all, no pain no gain, right? And I didn't feel any pain.

My urologist came on the line and said, "Congratulations your PSA is 3.6, right about where it should be."

What a sense of relief! I hadn't seen 3.6 in years. Even my earliest PSA readings were in the high threes. This was cause for celebration. I called my family and friends, shared the good news and took my wife out to dinner.

Six months later I was disappointed. I was expecting another 50% drop, but the reading was 3.3. It was 'technically' a drop, but why so little? Was this an indication that I was at the nadir (the bottom)? If so, that could spell trouble, as I had read somewhere that the lower the nadir, the better are your chances for long-term cure.

I called my radiation oncologist, Dr. Rossi at Loma Linda. He explained that I had nothing to be concerned about. Post radiation treatment PSA drop is never a straight line. It can be a "roller coaster ride," he explained. He told me that it can plateau and it can even temporarily bump up, especially during the first two years following treatment, and, "Not to worry. If it will make you feel any better, retest your PSA in three months instead of waiting six." I did, and my next reading – 13 months after treatment ended – was 2.3. Yes! Cause for another celebration.

I decided to test again in three more months. Again, good news: it had dropped to 1.0. By October 2002, 22 months after treatment, my PSA had fallen to 0.8. "God is good," I thought. All's right with the world!

Following is a chart of my PSA from the end of treatment in December 2000 through October 2006.

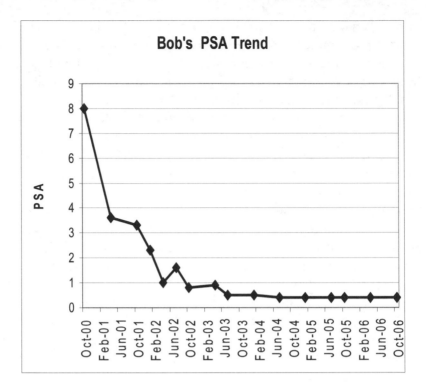

Bob's PSA Trend

Keep Your Prostate Quiet

In July 2002, I was scheduled for an annual physical including a PSA test. The previous reading was 1.0. My primary care physician had a substitute nurse that day. His regular nurse was on vacation, so things were a little out of sequence in his office. After the nurse measured my vital signs and ran the EKG, my doctor came in to finish the exam. As he slipped on his rubber glove, I asked him what he was going to do. "Your digital rectal exam," he said. "But you haven't drawn blood yet," I commented. "So what?" he replied.

I told him I had spent a long time researching PSA on the Internet and I learned anything that stimulates the prostate, such as orgasm, DRE, even riding a bicycle, could cause my PSA to spike resulting in a false reading.

"I've heard that," he said, "but I don't believe it."

I said, "OK, I'll bet you a buck my PSA will spike at least 30 to 50%." He said, "You're on."

Sure enough, my PSA came in at 1.6, and I wasn't alarmed. I repeated the PSA test – this time without the DRE – and the number was 0.8. I had convinced my primary care physician that the DRE must be done *after* blood was drawn for PSA, and I had won a buck. Life was getting better.

Later my PSA would reach a nadir in the 0.4 range, where it has remained for the past couple of years.

Other Changes in My Life

My life has changed in other ways. I maintained my increased exercise regimen and now exercise (run and workout) six days a week. I feel healthier and stronger than I have in years. Although my diet is not perfect, I find myself eating a generally healthier and more balanced diet as a result of the coaching from Stella, the nutritionist I met on my first day of treatment.

Many of the couples we met through proton treatment have become close friends. We exchange e-mails, phone calls and even travel and stay at each other's homes.

Advisory Council

In addition to maintaining contact with patients that I met during treatment, I stayed in touch with Dr. J. Lynn Martell, Vice President of Advancement for LLUAHSC, Loma Linda University Adventist Health Science Center, the umbrella organization for the University and Hospital. I didn't know much about his responsibilities at the time, other than the fact that he was involved in fund raising to support Proton therapy research and other programs at the Medical Center and University.

Shortly after I returned home, I wrote a letter to Dr. Lyn Behrens, CEO of all Loma Linda operations, acknowledging her and the staff for creating an unparalleled healing experience. The letter follows:

December 31, 2000

Dr. Lyn Behrens Pres. CEO
Loma Linda University Medical Center
11234 Anderson Street
P.O. Box 2000
Loma Linda, CA 92354

Dear Dr. Behrens,

I have just experienced a life-changing event. On December 21, 2000, I completed my proton beam treatment (PBT) treatment at LLUMC. Two months of exhaustive research led me to LLUMC, and to a prostate cancer treatment modality that I believe saved my life.

I had read much about PBT, so there were not many surprises with the systems and treatment once it began on October 26th. What did come as a pleasant surprise was the extraordinary compassion, care, concern, and professionalism I experienced and observed while undergoing my treatment.

I am 57 years old and have traveled the world as a senior executive for a Fortune 500 company. I have met people in the service professions, including the medical profession, in many parts of the world. Never have I experienced anything remotely close to the kind of treatment I received at LLUMC over the past two months.

There is something mystical, if not magical going on at LLUMC. Something very special and indeed, very spiritual is going on there. It all begins with the people, and not just with the medical staff.   It includes the finance, administration, social workers, receptionists, and others.

Patients at LLUMC get the feeling that everyone there sincerely cares about them. People there appear to be dedicated to doing their absolute best to treat the whole patient.

I have lived my entire life within a 60-mile radius of the self-proclaimed epi-center of medical research and excellence in the world, Boston, Massachusetts. I have availed myself of services at some of the finest hospitals in this region. The Boston medical community could learn volumes from LLUMC about the manner in which medical care should be delivered.

I would like to acknowledge a few of the people whose extra efforts and talents warrant special recognition. Dr. Carl Rossi and Sharon Hoyle - - what a team! I believe that the best gift one human being can give another is their time. These individuals gave my wife and me the time we needed to get our questions answered and to feel confident that we were getting the best medical attention available. If you could clone these two special people and place them in hospitals around the planet, you would revolutionize medical care as we know it.

Ed Schultz is a humble, hard working, and exceptionally competent manager who gives the patient great confidence in his technical knowledge and dedication to his work. He is serious about his work, yet possesses a sense of humor that relaxes both the staff and the patients. I was blessed to have been able to spend time with Ed learning about the technology, which I plan to share with prospective patients on the East Coast.

I would like to acknowledge the technicians in Gantry 3, beginning with Tim Holmes, an individual whom I would propose to be the model for this position. Tim has a presence, an attitude, and level of confidence, a sense of humor, and a manner that puts the patient at ease and convinces him that he is in the best hands.

Other special people in this area are Nick, Mark, and Barbara. Their jobs are not easy. Many aspects of their jobs are repetitive and downright unpleasant. Yet these folks come to work every day with a smile on their faces. Each patient feels important, respected, and well treated.

Gerry Troy, the untiring and totally dedicated social worker managed to convince even an engineer like me that the healing process is significantly enhanced when the patient feels a sense of community and support. Gerry consistently went out of his way to provide that measure of community, spiritual, and social support that truly communicated LLUMC's philosophy of "making man whole." Heather also did much to support this process and her efforts are much appreciated.

Dr. J. Lynn Martell epitomizes what a healing institution should be. He devotes countless hours giving of his time and talents; is continuously upbeat and optimistic; and is always there if you need him. His impact on patient morale is immeasurable.

While I did not spend a lot of time with these folks, I would also like to pass on my thanks and appreciation to Steve, the dosimetrist, Mary Lou the receptionist, Stella the nutritionist, Durlene the receptionist, Nancy, who filled in at Gantry 3, and other administrative folks including Marla, Michella, Maria Lordis, and even the people who handle billing and insurance who do their jobs with professionalism and pride.

All this, in my opinion, reflects on the management and administration of this outstanding institution.

For several years I consulted to companies in helping them learn and institutionalize the concepts of Total Quality Management. In the process of doing this, I became a true believer in the axiom that "management creates 'the system' and people work in 'the system.'" If management does a good job creating and improving the system in which people work, then the people will respond. You and your staff, Dr. Behrens, have done a magnificent job creating 'the system' at LLUMC. We, the patients are the beneficiaries.

God bless you, your staff, and the wonderful people at LLUMC for the exemplary work you are doing to set the world standard for medical excellence and care.

I know I speak for the other patients who were treated along with me, in expressing our sincere thanks and gratitude for the exceptional work that was done on our behalf. We wish you and all the wonderful people at LLUMC a very happy, healthy, holy, and bountiful New Year.

Sincerely,

Robert J. Marckini

C: Ms. Yoly Magana, Dr. James Slater, Dr. Jerry Slater, Dr. Lynn Martell, Mr. Norman McBride

In return I received a letter from Dr. Behrens humbly thanking me for taking the time to document my experience and for acknowledging the hard working people at Loma Linda.

About a month later, Dr. Martell sent me a letter inviting me to become a member of the Loma Linda University Medical Center Proton Treatment Center (PTC) International Advisory Council. The Council's mission is "To bring health, healing, and wholeness to those persons with cancer and other diseases through the clinical application of proton radiation." Council members are asked to be *Ambassadors* in enhancing strategic global outreach; *Counselors* in informing people, patients, and medical professionals, of the advantages of proton therapy; *Advisers* in developing educational programs for the public; *Advocates* for the Center in its clinical and basic research programs; and *Supporters* of the Center in identifying and generating financial resources to support the Center and its research efforts.

I willingly accepted and have been actively participating in Council activities ever since. As a member, I have been privileged to hear from Dr. Behrens, Ruthita Fike, Dr. James Slater, and Dr. Jerry Slater about their vision for the Medical Center, their plans and expectations for improving the precision of proton beam delivery, and the almost limitless applications of proton technology for treating numerous diseases for which there is no cure today.

As a Council member, I had the opportunity to tour the neonatal unit at this incredible medical institution, and see the extraordinary work being done to save the lives of countless babies who came into this world with severe, life-threatening birth complications. LLUMC, I learned, pioneered infant heart transplants and other leading edge neonatal medical technologies.

What struck me during the tour of the neonatal unit was the extraordinary care and compassion shown by the staff for the tiny patients entrusted to their care. This is the institution that created news with "Baby Fae," the little girl who received the heart of a baboon in 1984.

LLUMC has done more infant heart transplants than all hospitals in the world combined. To be connected with this institution in any way is an honor. To be a member of the PTC Advisory Council, promoting proton therapy, and supporting research and capital program funding has been a gift, for which I am truly thankful.

I am privileged to serve on this board with such people as Ken Venturi (golf professional and TV celebrity), John Raynolds (President and CEO National Peace Garden Foundation, former CEO Outward Bound), Phillip Livdahl (former Deputy Director of Fermilab and Chief Physicist on the LLUMC Proton Program), Ambassador Joseph Verner Reed (Under Secretary General of the United Nations), John Ebin (Commercial Developer and Philanthropist), Jim Tuggey (Marketing Executive and retired U.S. Army Colonel), Dr. Arnd Hallmeyer (German Physician), Doug Ayer (Venture Capitalist), John Butterfield (Retail Market Executive), Dr. Roy Butler (Retired Norwich University Professor), Dr. Jerry Klein (Scientist and Professional Photographer), Bill Vancil (Media Executive/Author), Steve Cohan (Media Executive), Gary Culpepper (Contractor/Developer), Paul Krauss (Management Consultant), Bill Linko (Inventor/Business Leader), Jerry Slakoff (Marine Surveyor), Ed Rosenberg (Financial Consultant), and several others.

This group meets twice yearly and focuses primarily on raising funds for proton therapy research, a cause to which I have become totally committed.

Invitation to Speak at Public Hearing in Hampton, Virginia

In mid 2005, I received a call from Dr. William Harvey, President of Hampton University in Hampton, Virginia. Hampton University is a progressive 6,200-student institution, founded in 1868, and today led by this dynamic visionary. It is located in a picture-postcard setting on 250 acres, with beautiful buildings and breathtaking grounds surrounded by water on three sides. It boasts the first medical physics program in the state of Virginia and the only one nationally at an historically black college.

They were holding a public hearing there to gain community support for a Proton Treatment Center. Dr. Harvey had done his homework. He had researched the technology well, brought in a top-notch physicist, aligned himself with a local oncology group, persuaded the community to donate the land, and gained the support of the Mayors of all the surrounding communities. The proton facility will be 96,000 square feet in size and will cost about $133 million.

I was proud to share the podium with other speakers like Dr. Jerry Slater, Chairman of the Department of Radiation Medicine at LLUMC, Dr. Alan Thornton, Medical Director at MPRI (Bloomington, IN), the Mayor of Hampton, and Don Gothard, from Washington, MI.

Dr. Harvey said the facility would be important, medically, for the Commonwealth of Virginia, and would be an economic driver for the local community. He envisioned an entire medical institution growing out of the proton treatment facility.

Following is the text of my talk:

My name is Bob Marckini. I am a prostate cancer survivor and a proton therapy patient. I am pleased to be speaking today in support of the Hampton University Proton Therapy Institute.

Coincidentally, it was five years ago today, August 10th, 2000, when I received a phone call from my urologist. He said, "The biopsy results are in; you have prostate cancer." I didn't hear much of what he said after that, but when my wife and I visited his office a few days later, he told me that I was a perfect candidate for surgery, and he'd be happy to do it. All I would have to do is to bank four pints of blood over the next month and I'd be ready to go. The brachytherapist I met with next said I was the perfect candidate for radioactive seeds; and

138

the radiation oncologist told me I was the "poster boy" for External Beam Radiation Therapy. The good news was that I had alternatives. The bad news was that each of them had the potential for complications like blood loss and infection, or side effects like impotence and incontinence.

One thing for certain: I was <u>not</u> going to choose surgery. Why? Because my older brother did that, two years prior, and I saw what he went through: Blood loss (six pints), tubes, drains, catheters, a long recovery, and all that was followed by a complication that required additional surgery. Also, a close friend had chosen surgery and he suffered some pretty nasty side effects. So, I began my research.

I admit to being a "recovering engineer," and I buried myself in the technical details. I did all the conventional things: read books, searched the Internet, and met with specialists in each field.

But the heart of my research consisted of interviews with former patients from each treatment modality. I was most interested in side effects and quality of life issues. It was the incontinence that concerned me the most. I was 57 years old, and the thought of wearing diapers for the rest of my life frightened me to death.

I learned about proton therapy the way most proton patients do, from a former patient. What I heard was hard to believe: "Non-invasive, no pain, no blood loss, minimal side effects – if any – and cure rates as good as the 'gold standard,' surgery." It sounded too good to be true . . . and I thought, "Why would anyone undergo major surgery with all the associated risks and side effects, if this painless and effective treatment were available?"

I continued my research, and spoke with former patients who had undergone surgery, brachytherapy (seeds), conventional radiation, and proton therapy. Of all those with whom I spoke, it was the proton patients who were most enthusiastic – bordering on ecstatic – about their treatment. I interviewed 56 of them. And they confirmed what I heard from the first one. No pain, non-invasive, and minimal to no side effects. The bonus was hearing how they played golf or tennis every day and had a great vacation during their two months of treatment.

139

I flew to Loma Linda for an orientation tour and consult. And when I saw the technology first hand, and met the wonderful folks at Loma Linda, that sealed the deal. I began treatment in mid October and finished in December 2000.

My treatment was at 7:20 AM five days a week. Each treatment lasted just a few minutes. I was out of there at 7:40 and spent the rest of the day with my wife exercising, playing golf, tennis, or site seeing. We had a great two-month vacation.

Doctors measure PSA, a protein in the blood, as a relative indicator of the effectiveness of prostate cancer treatment. My pretreatment PSA was 8.0, twice the upper limit of the normal range. Following treatment, as predicted, my PSA began to fall. Today, five years later, my PSA is 0.3 and I have experienced no permanent side effects. The quality of my life hasn't changed at all. I couldn't have asked for better results.

While in treatment five years ago, I made new friends . . . and, there is something stronger and deeper about friendships you make when you share a common bond, like prostate cancer. I was also struck by the type of men who were traveling there from all over the world for proton treatment. They were physicians, scientists, engineers, lawyers, physicists, college professors, and successful businessmen . . . all intelligent, analytical types who made decisions based on data. This made me feel good about my proton decision.

My new friends and I decided to form a club, so that we could keep in touch and compare notes as we continued our healing journey. We also wanted to maintain our connection with Loma Linda. The psychosocial programs there, combined with their extraordinarily caring attitude, created a wonderful, healing environment . . . and we didn't want to let that go. I volunteered to lead the group, which I named, "The Brotherhood of the Balloon." The word of our group's formation leaked out, others asked to join . . . and we grew larger.

Today, we have 2,100 members in 50 states and 17 countries. We have a website with our member database, a discussion board and many other features, including more than a hundred testimonials written by former patients. We have special projects to help members in various ways and we publish a monthly Newsletter. We promote proton therapy, both through our website, and by providing members with Power Point presentations to take on the road. On any given day, we have members around the world speaking at Lions' Clubs, Rotary Clubs, church and community meetings, and at men's prostate cancer support groups. Our reference list consists of dozens of former patients who welcome calls and e-mails from those who are evaluating treatment options and want to hear first hand about proton treatment.

In addition to providing support to our members, and promoting proton therapy, we have recently come to realize that we, who benefited from this extraordinary technology have an obligation to give something back to the institution that saved our lives, and the quality of our lives. To that end, we work to both refer patients to Loma Linda and to raise money for proton therapy research. To date, our group has referred more than 1,200 patients, and has raised more than $2.5 million for proton therapy research.

And we see this as just the beginning. As more Proton Treatment Centers are built, and more and more people discover the healing power of the proton beam, we see our group having much more impact on raising people's awareness of this technology, and bringing in significant funding for proton therapy research.

I thought when I received that phone call on August 10th, 2000 – five years ago today – that it was the lowest point in my life. Little did I know, that later I would consider that diagnosis to be one of the best things that ever happened to me.

My whole perspective on life and what's important in life has changed; I've had the opportunity to make new and wonderful friends; I've had the opportunity to discover Loma Linda, an extraordinary medical institution, with some of the most competent and dedicated people in the world; and it has given me the privilege of leading a support group and being a part of 2,100 people's lives, the overwhelming majority of whom have had their cancers cured, and the quality of their lives preserved.

Picture this: You are diagnosed with cancer. Your doctor encourages you to do major surgery and announces the possibility of blood loss, infection, and the high probability of impotence and incontinence. Next, imagine you discover a treatment that involves no invasion of your body, no blood loss, no infection, and significantly fewer side effects, if any. You would feel the weight of the world lifted from your shoulders. That's what happens with proton patients. That's what happened to me. And that's the experience of the other 2,100 members of our organization and the tens of thousands of patients who have been treated with proton therapy.

While at Loma Linda I met numerous people who benefited from proton treatment including Jennifer, a young woman who had a malignant tumor behind her eye. Her doctors said she was untreatable because of the tumor's location. It is now ten years after her proton therapy, and she's doing fine. I also met Daniel, a young man who had a tumor wrapped around his brain stem, diagnosed when he was 12 years old. After some surgery, doctors told his parents they couldn't get it all, and there was nothing more they could do. That was eight years ago. Proton therapy worked for him too. Today he's a junior in college and he's doing fine.

Proton beam therapy is an extraordinary technology – one that must be shared with the world. I can never thank Dr. Jerry Slater enough for what he and his team did for me at Loma Linda. And as long as I'm alive, I will do whatever I can to promote proton therapy.

Virginia should count itself fortunate that Hampton University is proposing to establish a Proton Therapy Center. Proton therapy has made a tremendous, positive impact on my life and the lives of the other members of my group. For the sake of the many patients who could benefit from proton therapy, I very much hope that you will approve the Hampton University Proton Therapy Institute. Thank you.

My Current Status

Prior to treatment, my PSA was 8.0 and my Gleason score was 3+2=5 from one pathology lab and 3+3=6 from another. There was no palpable tumor by DRE, so my cancer stage was labeled T1c.

Today, six years later, my PSA has leveled off at 0.4 and I am experiencing no side effects whatsoever. If anything, my health and physical condition are better than before treatment. My wife and I have continued the exercise regimen we began six years earlier at the Loma Linda Drayson Fitness Center. And, while our diet isn't perfect, it has been heavily influenced by our initial meeting with Stella, the LLUMC nutritionist, and continued contact with my friends at Loma Linda, who follow the Seventh-day Adventist diet and lifestyle. Adventists live as much as ten years longer than the rest of us, and they are generally much healthier years. A study funded by the U.S. National Institute on aging reported on this in the November 2005 issue of *National Geographics* Magazine.

My diet is low in animal fats, processed meats, beef, pork and lamb, as well as dairy products; I regularly drink soymilk and pomegranate juice; I have increased the number of daily servings of fresh fruits and vegetables; and I have increased my daily intake of water.

I exercise six days a week, alternating weight training with aerobics using a *Stair Stepper* or treadmill. I was slightly overweight prior to treatment, have worked to lose 12 pounds, and am currently at my ideal weight.

I take daily vitamins and supplements to support my health. These include lycopene, saw palmetto, vitamins E, D, and C, selenium, 81-grain aspirin, lecithin, and psyllium fiber.

CHAPTER 12

The Brotherhood of the Balloon

"We cannot become what we need to be by remaining what we are."
-- Max Depree

A Simple Beginning

Toward the end of treatment, my six new friends and I agreed that we would stay in touch with each other in order to continue our friendship and share information about our post treatment journey. I prepared a memo on my laptop computer to document this special occasion.

Members of this new fraternity willingly provided their information, returned the form to me, and the *Brotherhood of the Balloon* was born.

I had unknowingly left a couple of extra copies of the memo in the treatment waiting room. And, to my surprise, the next morning we had three new members, with a request for more memo-forms from the receptionist.

Following is the memo I sent to my six friends:

MEMO

TO: The Brotherhood of the Balloon   cc Dr. Carl Rossi
         ("BOB")   Sharon Hoyle
FROM: Bob Marckini   Ed Schultz

DATE: December 15, 2000

SUBJECT: <u>Sharing Information</u>

      I have spoken to a few of the guys who were treated in the October-December, 2000 timeframe about keeping in touch in the coming months and perhaps years. Seeing that we all have something in common, it seems to make sense that we stay in touch and share information about our progress.

      My thinking is that we could share information on our PSAs, side effects, etc. We could make ourselves available to each other to discuss problems or questions that might arise. We could also perhaps make ourselves available to other guys with prostate cancer who are dealing with the trauma that we experienced when we were diagnosed not so long ago.

      I suggest that we use e-mail as the primary vehicle for communication; however, if we all have each other's telephone number we can use the phone as well.

      I will volunteer to collect, summarize, and forward the information if you send it to me.

      If you are interested in participating in this communication process, please fill in the information below and return it to me before I leave on December 22nd, or provide it via e-mail, phone, or regular mail. If you don't know some of the information, or do not wish to share it, just fill in your name and e-mail address.

Thank you and good luck.

Name: _____   E-Mail: _____

Address: _____

Phone: _____   Treatment end date: _____

Age: _____   Pre treatment PSA: _____

Gleason Score _____   T- Score: _____

If you have any other suggestions for this communications process, please let me know.
Bob

When Gerry Troy and Dr. Martell heard about our "little group," they immediately saw something that I wouldn't see for months. They recognized that, while LLUMC psychosocial programs worked well at the medical center during the eight weeks of treatment, things changed dramatically when patients left to go home to their normal routine.

Both saw the *Brotherhood of the Balloon* as a natural extension of a process that began within the medical center, one that was totally consistent with LLUMC's mission. As a result, and unbeknownst to me, Gerry and Lynn became our marketing agents, talking up the BOB at every opportunity.

At a hospital patient Christmas party on the Monday before we left, Gerry announced that I had formed a new support group, and anyone interested in joining should see me.

The response surprised me. A few days later, when my wife and I left for home, we had 19 members of the *BOB*. I remember saying to my wife, "This was intended to be a small, private group of guys who just wanted to keep in touch . . . I suppose a few more won't matter. After all, the more, the merrier! But how could I possibly coordinate communications between 19 men from different locations around the country?"

A Life of Its Own

The word continued to spread at LLUMC after we left for home, mostly thanks to Gerry Troy and Dr. Lynn Martell. More and more patients wanted to join *The Brotherhood of the Balloon*. Each month Gerry would send me an envelope with a stack of sign up sheets filled out by patients I had never met. Now I was beginning to feel some pressure to turn this thing into something other than a secret men's club.

Within weeks I was receiving phone calls from former patients who had heard of our organization and wanted to join. I began mailing out sign up sheets from home and taking down member information over the phone.

The *Brotherhood of the Balloon* ("BOB") was taking on a life of its own. By December of 2001 our membership had grown to 282. Year-end 2002 saw membership at 736. Today we have almost 3,000 members from all corners of the earth. There seems to be no end to our growth.

We have members in Germany, Puerto Rico, Singapore, Australia, Great Britain, Ecuador, Guam, Saipan, Palau, China, Canada, Italy, the Bahamas, the Philippines, Venezuela, and many other locales. And members come from all walks of life including farmers, business leaders, physicians, scientists, educators, media personalities, professional athletes, clergy, engineers, bankers, lawyers, commercial pilots, stock brokers, sports celebrities, ambassadors, and judges.

Newsletter

The *BOB Tales* Newsletter is my primary communications vehicle with members. We started publishing the BOB Tales in mid 2001 and haven't missed a month since. I remember wondering if I could find enough relevant and substantive material to fill a newsletter on a monthly basis. As it has turned out, each month I have three or four times as much information as I can use in these publications.

Members from all over the world send articles and publications on subjects that may be of interest to our members, particularly related to the latest developments in prostate cancer awareness, detection, and treatment. I often abstract the articles and share them with members.

Every month we report on the status of new member additions; member feedback; the Featured Member of the month; prostate cancer prevention, detection, and treatment news; BOB member reunions; news from the major proton treatment centers; how we are doing on our mission to support each other, promote proton therapy, and give something back; health and nutrition suggestions and tips; and some humor to brighten their day.

Two members provide monthly articles to educate our members on timely issues. Dr. Roy Butler continuously reads, abstracts and reports on the latest developments in prostate cancer diagnosis and treatment. Renowned health educator Chuck Cleveland reports monthly on diet and lifestyle issues and tips that may help prevent prostate cancer and other cancers, as well as prevent a recurrence of cancer.

Support Group Meeting Notes

Many things have stimulated interest in our organization. The BOB is frequently discussed at the well-attended Wednesday night support group meetings at Loma Linda. 'Newbies' are anxious to stay in contact with those of us who have been through it.

The second factor stimulating interest in the BOB had to do with the informative and entertaining Wednesday Night Support Group meeting notes. These notes were initially published by Cal Jones, the Deputy District Attorney for San Bernardino County, who regularly attended support group meetings long after his treatment ended. With an excellent working knowledge of proton treatment technology and a gift for writing, Cal volunteered to take notes at the meetings and send them to me for distribution to BOB members. He did a wonderful job capturing the spirit, the humor, the emotion, and the camaraderie of the meeting. People who have "graduated" could now stay connected with the Loma Linda "family" through these meeting notes.

Following is an example from the July 18, 2001 meeting.

__Memories from the Wednesday Night Support Group Meeting__

July 18, 2001

- **Second Place Technology ~ Big Bucks for Investors?**
- **Precious Moments in the Pod ~ a Time to Reflect**
- **Salvage Radiation Therapy after Surgery**

Fairly crowded again. Gerry started off with jokes... he said some were from BOBs. He apparently gets quite a few... reads only some. He had a big smile on his face when he passed along one in particular: "How do lawyers sleep? [answer:] They lie on one side; and then on the other." Lots of people laughed... probably thought it funny; but I just had to stare at everyone because I figure most everyone sleeps that way... so what's the big deal! Oh well, I guess as one gets older that not all jokes are easy to grasp. He told more ... called them "lawyer jokes" for some reason, but they were all stale and,

---

besides I had heard them all anyway. When I heard them, however, they were called "social worker jokes" and "engineer jokes"… most were funny too, when I heard them the first time; but I won't bore you with Gerry's versions.

Then Gerry told us about an article that newbie *John (BOB)(the majestic and prestigious Brotherhood of the Balloon)* brought in to share: it is an article on Varian Medical Systems, Inc. [stock symbol: VAR …probably NYSE … selling around $71/s]… suggesting it is a good investment ploy… looks like a "bio-tech" firm. Anyway, the interest apparently stems from the fact that Medicare is approving payout increases… now paying twice as much for IMRT (Intensity Modulated Radiation Therapy) as for conventional radiation therapy… and that opens the door a lot wider for IMRT systems to be implemented across the U.S. It costs a whole lot less to build an IMRT facility as opposed to a proton beam facility, for sure. Anyway, the Varian company sells more than half of the IMRT systems in the U.S… and the article from the Investors Daily of June 16, 2001, projects that Varian's earnings will increase by 26% in one year, and another 19% in 2002.

Now, we all know that IMRT is reputedly very, very good… a very high-tech, conformal radiation system… a couple of people at the Wednesday Night Meeting have researched IMRT quite a bit and have reported to us that the scientific and medical communities are in substantial agreement: it is "almost as good as proton beam therapy!" And given the added fact that an IMRT facility costs a mere small fraction (less than $2 million) of what a proton beam facility would cost (maybe $150 million+ now), you can anticipate that many hospitals are going to convert to IMRT in the next few years. Varian has some competition, however… better research this idea if you are interested.

John (BOB 12/00) from Nevada started us off with some "veteran" news: four months post treatment psa was down to 2.9 ng/ml. That's a drop of 70%+ from his going-in numbers, psa 10.9, GS 7. John adds he feels "wonderful" and he looked it too… full of vim, enjoying a trek to California to see a new grandchild… clearly looking forward to many more years.

Another vet *Jack (BOB 5/01)* stopped in to report he had just got back from a 6600 mile motorcycle trip across and around the U.S. in the past six weeks since he completed his PBT. Jack says he has noticed "minimal side effects" despite many days of long hours on the motorcycle… trying to stay ahead of thunderstorms and otherwise just trying to move down the road, free as a bird it would seem.

Our real veteran, **Lt. Col. (ret) Bill** was again in attendance… he was busy with the cookies, of course, but paused with excitement to share his latest psa report: "hot off the press," he shouted… and he waved above his head a computer printout of his entire psa history… starting in 1993 with a 3.0, then it rose to 9.0+ in 1999… then Bill tried a concoction called Noni-Juice… took a quart of it over a week or so and the psa dropped drastically to 5.0! But I do not think it stayed there or maybe it was that it just did not go any further down… so Bill sought more traditional treatment and opted for conformal proton beam therapy. Bill reports his psa is now consistently 2.0 or a little below. Bill always has a joke to tell: a cop saw a woman driving in a convertible down the road… she was also knitting. So the cop pulled up along side and shouted to her "pullover"; at which the woman quickly retorted, "no, it's a scarf." Hey, it was funny hearing Bill tell it… what can I say. Bill left out his usual Viagra stories… we'll catch up on those other stories of Bill's next time. He visits us usually once a month. Newbies and grads alike enjoy Bill… he helps us all realize how vital humor is in keeping this entire journey in perspective.

One of Bill's favorite fans is *Joel (BOB)* who announced his good-byes tonight. Yep, Joel graduated. He says the ride so far… coming here for treatment, meeting so many people, dealing with all the new things… the feeling of community, etc,… all this has left Joel with so many memories, and memories similar to those he has of another emotional trip in his life: his service in Viet Nam. Both trips have left Joel with a feeling for how precious life is, for sure. Then… all along in both trips, he met new people, got to know them as friends and know them actually better than most relatives, and then he is now leaving just as he left "Nam"… probably never to see these new friends again… he has not seen his soldier buddies either. Except indirectly through his friend "Browny," whom Joel has told us about in the past few weeks. Remember, Browney is Joel's friend in Washington who served in the 10th Mountain Division in WWII… and now has reunited with two of his Army buddies who served in the same unit because Joel happened to strike up conversations with fellow patients in the corridors on level B. The latest on Browny, of course, is that he is still being considered for proton therapy that promises to extend his life significantly. Browny has been diagnosed with terminal cancer of some sort… anyway, we have all been pulling for Browny and I guess we will have to wait more to find out the rest of this story. Hopefully, Joel will keep us posted. Joel says he has felt "guilty" about calling home and reporting that all has been going so well... feeling fine, etc. Well, it really has been a breeze for Joel... but his buddies at work have had to knuckle under and work harder while Joel has been down here vacationing... er, I mean getting proton beam therapy. Joel reminds us that the time in the pod is one of "precious moments"... some time to reflect alright... like Joel explained that he often recalled seeing a sign from the freeway "Nevada Bob's." Joel thought about that sign in the pod often, apparently... he figured that the **BOB (the Brotherhood of the Balloon)** just had a Nevada chapter, and that it had established an outpost in California... but "they misspelled the sign." Joel finally stopped in the store and discovered it was a golf accessories shop. I do not know if Joel realized it, but it is also for sale... been going through bankruptcy for several months. In short, good news for golfers maybe...but just a pod memory to Joel. The mind sure does wander in that pod, alright: everyone in the room could identify with this story of Joel's.

Yoly Magaña dropped by to say hello. Yoly is the Executive Director of the Radiology Department. She is the one who supervises the non-doctor personnel and makes sure that the "Loma Linda Magic" is tuned-up and working as it should. Actually, I hear that she gets the job done by carefully selecting and training the employees... then just lets them be themselves... the "magic" naturally follows and is not taught or acquired. Momentarily she also has much on her mind due to two separate hospital inspection organizations being present throughout the hospital... poking around all corridors and asking questions of employees. I happened to have noticed a recent article that pointed out that MGH in Boston and Johns Hopkins in Baltimore were the nation's "top-rated" hospitals... so I asked Yoly what it takes to be considered so highly rated. She says she isn't sure, but she is looking into it. Someone in the audience interjected that the rating is not done by patients, "that's for sure!" ...that it is done by "peer" groups of doctors, at least certain doctors with the most political clout. It will be interesting, perhaps, what Yoly does find out in this regard... I will ask her again when she comes officially to our meeting to be our speaker.

Incidentally, that reminds me that Dr. James Slater and Dr. Rossi and Dr. (PhD) Miller (Chief Physicist) are also scheduled to be speakers in the near future. Each of them probably has some idea about how to answer such a question, too.

Several newbies in the crowd... all enjoying the generally "favorable" veteran and graduate reports. Stan from Colorado just started last Monday... psa around 4.5 and GS "6-7". Stan says a friend told him of "this place called Loma Linda" so he came here! It seems like it is that simple, doesn't it?

David (BOB) is a newbie with quite a story... started about six years ago with a psa of 7.0 and a GS 6. And with a radical prostatectomy... that is, SURGERY, the "gold standard". Well, all appeared fine until six months ago... the psa has been rising. David comes from a family that has a history of PCa, so David is not the type to wait around to see what can happen... he knows. He says that after his surgery, he did keep researching and learning... and with what he now knows, he would have chosen PBT..., but he only discovered PBT after the fact. He is here now for salvage treatment.

I recently was talking to one of the physicians, and he pointed out that in cases of surgery that need salvage radiation therapy, in the majority of such cases, the cancer is still "local" and focused in the prostate bed (area where the prostate gland had been). So radiation therapy can be very effective in such cases. I heard that about 5% of proton beam PCa patients routinely treated at LLUMC are former surgery patients who had rising PSA after treatment. The key in such cases, however, is not to wait too long... "watchful waiting" or just ignoring the problem is a no-no according to the doctors ... and our newbie David too. The main point, however, is that quite a few men here for proton beam therapy have had surgery with a still rising psa.

David is talkative, insightful, and a newbie only in the sense that he is new to PBT. David is really a veteran in light of all his knowledge and the amount of time he has spent on this journey. We'll hear more from David, I am sure.

A newbie stood up suddenly... "to defend Stella". Yep, to think some people tend to make fun of Stella's advice! Remember, Stella Jones is the nutritionist... no vegetables, just meat, no seeds, no spices... no roughage... I do not recall all her rules. Anyway, this newbie stood up to warn us all that there really can be a danger in ignoring Stella's dietary rules. For example, this newbie with only eight (photon?) treatments to go, ate potato skins and broccoli and ended up *"feeling like he was passing razor blades."* Now, that could be an annoying feeling, if you ask me!! In short, his message is that "you better pay attention to Stella" or you could end up with your "tail pipe hurting." I didn't catch this newbie's name... I think he has another week to go, however, and next week I suspect he will have a few more choice bits of colorful wisdom to pass (oops, that is probably an inappropriate way to put it).

Gary from Texas is a newbie… added his hello's. I didn't get Gary's numbers… I think mainly because he emphatically introduced himself as an "listener" and not a talker. Gary says he learns more that way. Kind of made everyone pause and think for a second… like a moment of silence in a church. Anyway, Gary did tell us something interesting about himself and this journey: Gary has been on Lupron for three years before deciding to opt for conformal proton beam therapy. Now, that is a record for anyone I have met at the Wednesday Night Support Group Meeting. We'll possibly hear more about hormone ablation therapy from someone who really knows in the next few weeks…. that is, if Gary will choose to talk a little more. Oh, by the way, Gary says he got "tired of it [the Lupron therapy]".

Dr. Lynn Martell reported that veteran *Roy (BOB 3/00)* phoned from back home in Vermont… sends greetings to everyone… and adds that he is going to meet with *Lloyd (BOB 1/01)*, also from Vermont, and they are going to attend a support group back there. Roy reports that the likely topic will be how PBT can be used advantageously for follow-up salvage treatment of those who have had surgery, but the psa continues to spook them. Liable to be a few more Vermonters out our way in the future.

A well-informed newbie from Iowa announced his hello… *Dick,* I believe is his name. Dick says he has a cousin named Doyle in Seattle who somehow steered him to Loma Linda. Dick says his story started a few years ago… psa 5.8, then after some antibiotics his psa was 4.9, then a biopsy ("benign")… then waited a year, and his psa was 6.83, but this time when he was given antibiotics, the psa went to 8.0+. So another biopsy (ouch!) and a Gleason score of 6. Dick just completed his eighth treatment. Dick also revealed that he is an M.D. … a retired anesthesiologist.

This is the second anesthesiologist that has been here in two weeks. And I think one or two other doctors that have been here as patients have also been anesthesiologists.

No poetry or songs tonight. And also no one yet has turned out to be a tap dancer (at least no one has admitted it). So the meeting ended "on time"… shorter than usual, for a change, but apparently still as inspiring because people hung around and continued their pet conversations, prying answers and bits of wisdom from one another and all the veteran proton beamers.

Cal has since retired, but the notes continue to this day, thanks to the efforts of volunteers who are often the wives of men in treatment.

New Sign-up Sheet

Now that we had gone "big time," the BOB needed an updated member application form. This document, which was typically distributed at the Wednesday night meetings, requested more detailed information than the first form.

Membership continued to grow. We were now attracting members from states all across the nation and from locations outside the U.S.

The information collected on these forms was summarized on a database and distributed monthly to each member by e-mail.

Brotherhood of the Balloon (BOB) Registration Form

We are an independent support group dedicated to providing information and support to former Proton patients; to help others discover proton treatment; and to give something back to LLUMC. Member benefits include access to other former patients; monthly newsletter; weekly notes from Wed. night meeting; access to our secure website (www.protonbob.com) including Member Database; news on the latest developments in preventing, detecting, and treating prostate cancer and recurrent prostate cancer; information about Proton Alumni Reunions; and much more.

Please fill out the following registration form for membership. Only name, address, and e-mail address are mandatory, but most members provide <u>all</u> the information. This benefits us, and others, in many ways.

Name: first_____ last_____wife's first name:_____

Address (street, city, state, zip, country or region)_____
_____

Phone: home_____work_____cell_____
E-mail Address: _____
(If you do not have e-mail, we will mail you hard copies of our Newsletters. But e-mail saves us mailing costs and gives you access to all BOB communications)

Have you ever been treated for prostate cancer before? (yes/no) _____

If so, by what method? _____

Treatment received (check all that apply): Proton__Photon___Hormones__

Treatment End Date (Estimate if not sure): Month _____Year_____

Age When Treated: _____ **Highest PSA before treatment:** _____

If treatment completed, please provide most recent PSA and date:
PSA_____; Date (mo./yr.)_____

What was your pretreatment Gleason Score? __**T-score** (if known): __

Was there a palpable (detectable) Tumor by DRE? (yes/no) _____

What is (or was) your profession? _____**Retired?** (yes/no)___

Medical Insurance Carrier: Primary _____; Secondary _____

OK to share your information with non-members who are evaluating treatment options? (yes/no) _____

How did you learn about Proton Treatment? _____
_____
_____
Comments: _____
_____

Something in Common

When I was conducting my due diligence for choosing a prostate cancer treatment option, I focused on speaking with patients, the 'customers,' and I learned much more from them than I did from the physicians, many of whom seemed to be 'pushing' their specialty. I especially sought out men whose cancer stage was similar to mine.

In designing the BOB application form, I made sure I captured enough information to be helpful to others in the future. I learned that not only do men like to talk with others of similar cancer stage, they often want to talk with someone of comparable age, profession, and sometimes even location.

Lawyers seem to like to talk with lawyers, clergy with clergy, physicians with physicians, and so on.

Dealing with prostate cancer all day can be a bit of a downer. So I try to lighten things up now and then when talking with recently diagnosed men. One day, when I was in a particularly giddy mood, I received a call from a gentleman who identified himself as a pilot. At that time, we had upwards of 50 pilots in our group, so I thought I'd have some fun with him:

"Would you like to speak with another pilot?" I asked.
"I'd love to." He replied.
"OK. Commercial or private?"
"Ah, private."
"Fixed wing or helicopter?"
"Are you serious? . . . uh, fixed wing."
"Piston engine or jet?"
"This is amazing," he said, "Piston."
"Single engine or twin?" I asked.
"Twin," he gasped. I could almost hear his jaw drop.
So I gave him the name of one of our members who flies a twin-engine piston plane.

Medical Insurance Help

Proton therapy costs more, primarily because of the capital investment needed to build a proton treatment facility. More than $100 million is typically required to purchase the particle accelerator and build a facility with multiple, hundred ton rotating gantries and computer control systems. They also require a large number of people to operate and maintain these complex systems.

Because proton therapy costs more than the alternative treatment options, some medical insurers (usually HMOs) deny coverage.

There has been a significant benefit in having the medical insurance provider question on our registration form. Occasionally an insurer will deny coverage for proton therapy, claiming it's 'too new,' or it's 'experimental,' forcing their insured customers to choose surgery, seeds, or conventional radiation.

However, if XYZ Insurance Company has already reimbursed one of our members in Dallas, and another Texas resident is denied by that same insurer, we know it, and we can provide this information to the individual whose request was denied. We have helped members turn around denials using this approach on several occasions.

We have put together an Insurance Strategy File, which contains game plans and tactics for appealing denied insurance claims for proton therapy. The file contains information on FDA approval for proton therapy, a list of 180 private insurers who cover proton therapy, and well thought out arguments for any type of denial. The Insurance Strategy File has helped dozens of our members win their appeals.

Our membership now has representation from all 50 U.S. states and 21 countries around the world. And members come from all walks of life including farmers, business leaders, physicians, lawyers, scientists, media personalities, sports celebrities, ambassadors, and judges. Adding even more credibility to the proton treatment process is the presence of urologists, physicists, and physician/cancer researchers in our ranks.

Counseling Men

As the word got out, through our membership and later our website, that I had done extensive research into the treatment options, I began receiving phone calls and e-mails from men who were diagnosed with prostate cancer. I gave willingly of my time, as I was once there myself, and others gave to me. Every day I receive a growing number of calls and emails, and they all start out pretty much the same way. "My name is Charlie, I'm 59 years old and I've been diagnosed with prostate cancer. My PSA is 5.2 and my Gleason score is 3+4 . . . ."

I admit to being biased in favor of proton treatment. Many of the men I counsel choose the proton option, not so much because I am 'selling' it, but because of my passion for the technology that comes across in our conversations. The extensive data now available proves that this non-invasive treatment works; it does so without pain, anesthesia, catheters, and risks of many of the other options; and with many fewer side effects and complications than the alternatives.

When people call or e-mail me, I just tell my story. I relate how important I feel it is to talk directly with patients who have chosen each of the options, and how difficult it was for me to get names, until I contacted Loma Linda.

I direct them to our website and encourage them to read the FAQs, the member testimonials, and the ten year peer-reviewed published study on proton therapy, as well as the fifteen year report. Then I send them two powerful documents: 1) a comprehensive University of Pennsylvania article by Dr. James Metz, which compares proton therapy to surgery and conventional, conformal radiation, and 2) the names of about fifty of our members who volunteer to communicate with those who are researching treatment options. Finally, I share with them what I learned during my own due diligence about the major treatment options, including the pros and cons of each.

I continue to learn more every day as our 3,000 members share with me the latest articles and information they find on prostate cancer prevention, diagnosis, and treatment.

One gentleman, a business leader in Rhode Island called me after he had made a decision to do IMRT in Florida. He was scheduled to have his procedure begin within four weeks. He had heard through a friend that I received proton therapy and was very happy with the results. We spoke several times. I shared the results of my research with him and put him in touch with the people at LLUMC. He flew out to the West Coast in his own plane and met with some of the medical staff. A week later he called to tell me he canceled his IMRT appointment and scheduled Proton Treatment in California.

Over the past six years I have spoken with literally thousands of people about my treatment – including a well known psychologist from Massachusetts, a pilot from Montana, a dentist from Tennessee, a developer from Minnesota, a venture capitalist from Connecticut, a foreign ambassador, a radio personality from Texas – they have all chosen the proton option, with very satisfactory results. Many of these men have become friends.

There is a large and growing fraternity of prostate cancer survivors who are proton 'graduates.' There is a special bond between us. And for some reason this is much different from the relationships former patients have within other treatment modalities. Is it the protons? Is it Loma Linda? I'm not sure. But I do know there is something special in that connection, and it works to the benefit of us proton graduates.

Unfortunately, I have come across some sad cases too. These usually had to do with individuals who, for various reasons, failed to have annual physical examinations or – believe it or not – had doctors who didn't believe in running routine PSA tests.

One instance I recall happened in May of 2001. The wife of a recently diagnosed prostate cancer patient called. She was doing research on treatment options for her husband and wanted to learn all she could about proton treatment from me. I asked my typical opening questions: What is your husband's age, his PSA, his Gleason Score, and is there a palpable tumor by DRE?

She told me he was 56 years old, his PSA was 37, his Gleason score was 10, and he had large tumors in both lobes of his prostate. My "knee-jerk" reaction was, "Surely this must have shown up in previous physical exams?" And she replied, "He's never had any physical exams. We don't believe in them. We prefer health food, meditation and yoga to conventional western medicine."

"Then how did you discover his cancer," I asked. She replied, "He couldn't urinate, so we went to the hospital emergency room where they discovered the tumors."

What is so sad about this case is her husband was a young man. Routine physical examinations and blood tests would have detected his cancer years before. At this stage, it may be too late. I wanted to tell her that the best advice I could offer was to have her husband get his affairs in order and prepare for the worst. But instead I told her that I was not qualified to offer any suggestions in this case; I gave her the names of two physicians, and suggested she discuss her husband's case with them.

Little did I know back on August 10, 2000, when I received the call in Nantucket notifying me of my diagnosis, that years later I would be leading an international support group and counseling men all over the world.

Our Mission

Over the years, our mission as a support group has evolved into three objectives: 1) To provide aftercare support, communications and education to members, 2) To help others discover proton therapy, and 3) To give back to the institution that saved our lives and preserved the quality of our lives.

In the more than six years since our founding, we have done well in all three areas.

Aftercare support, communications and education happens through our formal communications (monthly newsletters and support group meeting notes) and informal communications (reunions, emails, and telephone). Numerous special educational projects have been initiated to aid individuals with specific problems ranging from erectile dysfunction to medical insurance problems. Members without computers and e-mail access are "sponsored" by members who have Internet access, and hard copies of our correspondence are sent through the mail to our "e-mail-challenged" brothers.

We help others discover proton therapy through the special presentations our members deliver at community meetings, through newspaper and magazine articles written by members, and from thousands of one-on-one communications our members have with recently diagnosed men. Each year, our group routinely refers several hundred men to proton therapy – men who would otherwise have chosen surgery, seeds or some other treatment option.

Since the vast majority of our members were treated at Loma Linda University Medical Center, we focus our "giving back" efforts on contributing to proton therapy research there, primarily through the Dr. James Slater Endowed Chair for proton therapy research, which was initiated by *The Brotherhood of the Balloon*. To date, our members have contributed more than $2.5 million to LLUMC research programs, mostly through cash contributions and planned giving.

CHAPTER 13

A New Website
www.protonbob.com

"Use what talents you possess: the woods would be very silent
if no birds sang there except those that sang best."
--Henry Van Dyke

By early 2002, membership was growing at more than 30 new registrations per month, and our "manual" database, containing 22 pieces of information on over 300 members was becoming impossible to manage.

I engaged a small graphic design firm, Markus Design Group, to create a logo and establish a website for the BOB. The logo was perfect.

Next they developed a website that went far beyond my expectations in terms of layout, attractiveness, features, and ease of navigation. In addition to the standard Home Page, Frequently Asked Questions (FAQs), About Us, Privacy Statements, Helpful Links, and other standard features, they provided some unique and user-friendly features.

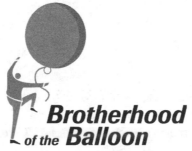

Password Protected

The site is split into two sections, one accessible to the general public, and the other password protected for members only. Prospective BOB members must be current or former proton patients. To become members, they visit our website home page, click on "Sign up," provide their data, including their own user name and password, and submit the information to me. I review it and either accept or reject the application.

Member List

All legitimate applications are accepted. Member information is now displayed on a comprehensive, interactive member database. Name, address, e-mail, phone numbers, age when treated, pretreatment PSA, Gleason Score, T-stage, specific treatment received, current PSA, occupation, medical insurance carrier, and more are all displayed in one database. At this writing, there are about 50,000 pieces of data displayed on our website member list.

With sorting capability, members can choose to rearrange the data and sort based on home state, age, PSA, Gleason Score, treatment received, medical insurance carrier, and other criteria.

Newsletter

The secure part of the website also contains my monthly newsletter, *BOB Tales*. The newsletter is located in the secure area because members' names and personal information are included in these publications.

Discussion Board

A discussion board was added in 2003. Members could post questions or comments on any subject related to their treatment and solicit responses from other members. Questions covered such subjects as side effects, medical insurance coverage, and life after proton treatment.

Proton Patient Testimonials

Member testimonials are the heart of the website. When I look back on the issues that most influenced my treatment decision, it was hearing from the 'customers,' the patients of each treatment modality. Their stories meant so much to me; *it was the single most important factor in my decision.* For this reason, I decided to ask some of our members to document their stories for my website. I would call this "Proton Patient Testimonials." Today there are 130 testimonials on www.protonbob.com.

This has turned out to be the most important link on my website. On dozens of occasions, I have heard recently diagnosed men say that they chose proton therapy largely as a result of reading these testimonials.

There are testimonials written by men from all walks of life, including, Warren Johns, an attorney who happened to be consulting to the Loma Linda University Medical Center Board when they were considering making the huge capital investment for the proton facility. He voted against it. Later, when he was diagnosed with prostate cancer, Warren became a beneficiary of proton therapy at Loma Linda. Today, fourteen years later, Warren is cancer free thanks to the healing power of the proton beam. He is now a strong proponent of proton therapy for prostate cancer.

Lots of physicians seem to gravitate to proton treatment. This alone is testimony to the efficacy of the technology.

Dr. Arnd Hallmeyer, from Berlin, Germany had a PSA of 436 when diagnosed in 2000. While working as a nurse in his early medical career, Dr. Hallmeyer assisted in performing radical prostatectomies. The invasiveness of those surgeries left an indelibly etched memory which, many years later, prompted him to search for a better alternative when diagnosed with prostate cancer. Today, he is cancer free and is leading a project to build a proton treatment facility in Berlin.

Dr. Terry Wepsic's testimony is compelling. Terry's situation is unique. Not only is he a physician, he is a pathologist, cancer researcher and professor of pathology. When people with credentials like his choose proton therapy, others sit up and take notice.

During his consult with Dr. Rossi at Loma Linda in early 2003, Terry looked at the doctor, and said, "I know you from somewhere." Dr. Rossi smiled and responded, "That's right. You were my pathology professor at Loyola."

Bob Reimer's testimonial is significant. Bob's PSA started rising rapidly in 1997. After ruling out infection, he was diagnosed with advanced prostate cancer, with PSA 61 and Gleason score 10. It doesn't get much worse than that. His doctor told him he probably had one to three years to live and he should go home, get his affairs in order, and prepare to die. That was almost ten years ago. Bob discovered Loma Linda and proton treatment. Today his PSA is 0.2; he is cancer free; and has experienced no side effects.

John Ebin is perhaps the only individual I know who did more research than I when diagnosed. John didn't settle for Internet searches and phone conversations. He wanted to see, touch, and feel each option. So he traveled the country, visiting the premier medical institutions, looking for the absolute best option for his prostate cancer.

I met John in mid 2002. We had dinner at the Four Seasons Hotel in Boston. John impressed me with his knowledge of all the major treatment options and with his probing questions about the option I believed in so strongly. After numerous follow-up conversations, John chose proton therapy and has had excellent results.

Dr. Roy Butler's testimonial is a 'must read.' Roy is the college professor I wish I'd had for organic chemistry. He's extremely intelligent, yet humble, and has a sense of humor that disarms and relaxes you. His knowledge of proton therapy and technology is second only to the good doctors and physicists at Loma Linda University Medical Center. His treatise, *The Patient Proton*, which can be found on my website is the best layman's perspective on proton technology I have found.

How did he acquire this knowledge? During treatment, he became so enamored with proton technology, he decided to "hang around" for a while after treatment ended. He arranged for a sabbatical from Norwich University in Northfield, Vermont so he could teach at the University of Redlands, a short distance from LLUMC. During that time, Roy studied proton therapy, interviewed the physicists and physicians at Loma Linda, and authored *The Patient Proton.*

Bill Vancil was treated in 2004. He used his treatment time as a way of reconnecting with his daughter, Tori Lou. She joined him during his treatment and they had an extraordinary time together. Bill later wrote a book, *Don't Fear the Big Dogs*, about this journey. It is a heartwarming story and it provides a good perspective on proton therapy.

Judge William Auslen, from Carlsbad, CA was our 1,000[th] member. He was treated more than ten years ago and has had excellent results according to his testimonial. Bill is a strong proton advocate and a regular contributor to proton therapy research.

Dr. Jerry Klein's story is also an excellent read. Jerry was one of the first six BOB members and the individual who recommended the establishment of the Dr. James Slater Endowed Chair for Proton Therapy Research. This endowed chair has been funded by the *Brotherhood of the Balloon* and is now supporting critically important proton therapy research.

Colonel (Retired) Howard J. "Jim" Tuggey wrote an inspiring testimonial. Jim was treated with protons in 1999 and today is cancer free with zero side effects. He has become an advocate for proton therapy promoting this modality worldwide. His website, www.prostateproton.com has influenced hundreds of men to choose proton therapy for their prostate cancer.

Alex Plummer's testimonial has been an inspiration to many, especially African American men, who are at 60% greater risk for prostate cancer. Alex lost his father to prostate cancer at age 53, and entered a deep depression when he received the news of his own diagnosis. His faith and his family helped him through the difficult times. His story appeared in *Guidepost Magazine*, and today Alex speaks to groups about prostate cancer awareness and early diagnosis.

Bill Hansell, a national leader in county government is President of the National Association of Counties. He was finishing treatment when I was being treated in 2000. I was impressed with his willingness to share his story with his community back in Athena, Oregon, by writing monthly stories of his treatment experience at Loma Linda for his local newspaper. Bill's testimony has helped many feel comfortable with proton therapy.

Ed Souder is a hero. He's a member of "The Greatest Generation," a World War II veteran, who suffered severe injuries from an artillery shell that exploded next to his jeep, killing his friends and leaving him near dead. His battle with prostate cancer was just a bump in the road. He believes God led him to Loma Linda and his faith sustains him to this day. His testimonial is inspiring.

Cal Jones was Deputy District Attorney for San Bernardino County. And, for a lawyer, a pretty nice guy! We became friends during treatment and remain so today. Cal is extremely knowledgeable about proton therapy and has written a comprehensive testimonial.

Members range in age from early 40s to early 90s. The senior citizen of our group is Charlie Einsiedler from Rhode Island. His story, on our website, is testimony to his engineering background, his tenacity, and his perseverance. He did considerable research, which included visiting premier medical institutions. And when his urologist suggested hormone therapy, Charlie refused, because he was too young for "chemical castration." Six years after treatment and 93 years young, Charlie still plays golf three times a week, but admits to "getting a bit tired" after 18 holes.

Three of the testimonials on our website were written by former surgery patients who had a prostate cancer recurrence. They are Charlie Rubin, David Leighton, and Bob Young. Their stories are compelling and are a chilling reminder that removing the cancerous gland from your body is not a guarantee of a cure. In fact, while I was at Loma Linda, I learned that about 5% of prostate cancer patients treated are former radical prostatectomy patients whose cancer returned after surgery.

All 130 testimonials provide value and insight to recently diagnosed men; they have been instrumental in leading hundreds to proton therapy.

Wednesday Night Meeting Notes

These were discussed earlier. This weekly communiqué has become an integral part of our support system. Archived notes are posted on the secure section of our website.

Photo Pages

A few months after establishing the website, we added three photo pages – later expanded to six – with pictures of Loma Linda, treatment gantries, local tourist attractions, and BOB members. Seeing the smiling faces of people undergoing cancer treatment helps dispel some of the myths people conjure up in their mind about the 'torture' of cancer treatment.

Website Traffic

Today, more than 6,000 people visit the website each month, representing 100,000 page hits. Average time per visitor is 12 minutes, a statistic that website analysts tell me, indicates we are holding their attention. Another way of looking at this: 6,000 visitors spending an average of 12 minutes means that our website is being visited for 1,200 hours every month.

CHAPTER 14

A Word About Medical Insurance

This subject is so important I felt a chapter should be devoted to it.

"You may never know what results come from your action. But if you do nothing, there will be no result."
                                                    -- Mahatma Gandhi

One More Difference Between Procedures

As you have seen in this book, there are many differences between prostate cancer treatment options. But there is one more important difference between proton treatment and all the other options – cost.

Cost of Surgery

Radical prostatectomies are performed in operating rooms. These are the same operating rooms that are used for appendectomies, tonsillectomies, heart by-passes, hernia repairs, and the like. In other words, these procedures are carried out in conventional hospital operating rooms that can be used for limitless surgical procedures.

Specialized equipment required for these procedures generally costs from tens of thousands to a few hundred thousand dollars and can be brought into the operating room.

A radical prostatectomy requires a surgeon, anesthesiologist, pathologist, surgical assistants, and follow up care by nursing staff and physician during the short hospital stay. Subsequent visits for catheter management and removal and consults are also part of the radical prostatectomy process.

All this costs money. But, once again, the procedure is done in a conventional operating room, and the cost of this facility is shared by all the other procedures performed there. Likewise the recovery room, the hospital room, the nursing staff, etc. arc all shared by a large patient population and a wide variety of medical procedures, all helping to keep the cost of these procedures down.

So, if a radical prostatectomy costs the medical insurer $25,000 (or even $35,000 to $40,000 at the more pricey centers of excellence), generally speaking, everybody is happy. The doctor and hospital earn a profit, as they should; the insurance company pays a reasonable amount for the procedure; and the patient pays nothing, or perhaps a small deductible on his policy.

Cost of the Other Treatment Options

Most of the other procedures are performed in similar facilities, with staffs that handle numerous other medical procedures.

Most forms of external beam radiation are done in conventional radiotherapy treatment facilities. Certain specialized devices are used to focus the beam and/or modulate radiation energy. In the case of IMRT for example, the price tag for specialized equipment is reported to be in the $1 million range. Again, this procedure is done in a conventional hospital setting, with staff that handles many other medical procedures and tasks.

In the case of conventional (X-ray) three-dimensional conformal radiation, patient work up and preparation (imaging, studies, interdisciplinary consultations, etc.) are similar, and thus costs for this portion of treatment are similar.

Brachytherapy and Cryosurgery may require some specialized equipment and instrumentation as well, but these procedures too can be performed in a conventional setting.

The bottom line: Specialized equipment capital costs for doing most of the above procedures are modest; and facilities, equipment, and personnel for these procedures are typically shared with other medical procedures. The costs, therefore, can be shared and thus maintained in a moderate range, allowing both hospital and physician to earn a profit and the insurer to pay a modest sum for the above procedures, reportedly in the $20,000 to $40,000 range per patient.

The situation with proton therapy is quite different.

Proton Treatment Facilities, Equipment, and Staffing

The capital investment to build a proton treatment facility is substantial. The facility at Loma Linda cost $100 million. Massachusetts General Hospital reportedly paid close to that for their facility, which has one less treatment gantry. MD Anderson spent $125 million to build their proton center, as did the University of Florida, in Jacksonville. The Midwest Proton Radiology Institute in Indiana spent about $40 Million to construct their proton treatment unit, but they built it around an existing cyclotron. Hampton University in Virginia has earmarked more than $180 million to build their proton treatment facility. The University of Pennsylvania plans to spend $144 million for their proton treatment center.

Why is the cost so high? Many reasons. First, the space requirement is significant. Considerable real estate is needed to house the particle accelerator and multiple treatment rooms. The cost of the very specialized cyclotron or synchrotron required to generate high speed proton particles is substantial. At Loma Linda, each treatment gantry is three stories high and weighs 100 tons. For safety reasons the entire facility is surrounded by 14 foot thick concrete and steel walls. Significant computer capacity, control and instrumentation are required to safely and precisely manage the proton beam.

A large staff is needed to manage the synchrotron or cyclotron during the treatment process and to do daily calibration and maintenance. Physicists and dosimetrists are required to plan and manage patient customized treatment protocols. Add to that the dedicated oncologists, case managers, nurses, and radiation therapists, and the cost of staff becomes significant. The Proton Treatment Unit at LLUMC requires a staff of about 80 people.

Loma Linda adds one more dimension, generally not seen elsewhere. The radiation treatment unit has assigned its own dedicated staff of social workers who focus on the psycho-social part of the healing process. This is a critical factor in LLUMC's stated mission, "To Make Man Whole."

The bottom line is this: It costs significantly more money to treat prostate cancer with proton therapy than by other treatment modalities. That's a fact of life.

What is the payoff for the patient? Very simply, it is quality of life. In some cases it is life itself. Proton beam therapy has been shown to cure 45 cancers and other diseases, including some that are untreatable by other means. And, in the case of prostate cancer, it can clearly be shown that there is less collateral damage to surrounding organs and tissue, and therefore side effects are significantly fewer than with any other option, short of watchful waiting.

Medicare and the overwhelming majority of private insurance companies, who recognize the efficacy of proton treatment and the value to the patient, willingly pay the higher price for this premium treatment. Some of the *low budget* medical insurers resist paying the higher cost for proton treatment, ostensibly because there are 'comparable,' lower cost options. This obviously causes considerable difficulty – not to mention anxiety – for the patient who chooses proton. The operative word, here, is *comparable*. Once the data is examined, it can quickly be learned that these treatments are not comparable.

The good news is that efforts are underway to reduce the cost of proton therapy:

- Treating patients around the clock spreads overhead costs over more patients and lowers costs.
- Using robotics to position the patient more rapidly and more accurately will allow higher patient throughput.
- The use of radiation sensitizers and desensitizers will improve patient throughput.
- The design of lower cost linear/laser proton accelerators will reduce capital requirements.
- Other studies underway will improve productivity and lower costs.

New proton treatment facilities are springing up all over the world. As knowledge increases, productivity will increase and cost will come down.

Medicare Pays

Our own (U.S.) Medicare system routinely pays for those over 65 who choose this procedure. Today, Medicare pays for about half the men treated for prostate cancer at Loma Linda. The remainder are covered by about 180 private medical insurers, such as Blue Cross Blue Shield, AARP, Aetna, Tricare, GEHA, Healthnet, and United Healthcare.

My medical insurer was Blue Cross Blue Shield of Massachusetts, and they were superb. The approval was given in 24 hours, no questions asked. I have been with Blue Cross Blue Shield for many years and have always been pleased with their coverage and service.

HMOs Are the Worst

Not all insurance companies readily reimburse for proton treatment. Some march to a different drummer. They seem to have the philosophy: If a lower cost option has been shown to be effective in treating the disease, than that is all we will pay for. And HMOs seem to be the worst offenders.

One problem I have with HMOs and other medical insurers that deny coverage for proton treatment is they are not being honest with the patient. Rather than saying, "We choose not to cover proton therapy because it is more costly than the alternatives," they claim, "Proton treatment is experimental," or it is "investigational," or "Proton treatment has not been proven to be superior to other forms of treatment."

To that, I say, "Look at the data." Or, even more important, talk to the thousands of patients who have been cured of their cancers, and have suffered minimal to no side effects. Compare them to the tens of thousands of men who are suffering debilitating side effects from the other forms of treatment. How can you put a price tag on that?

Proton beam therapy has been used to cure cancer for more than 50 years. It has been practiced in a hospital setting for more than sixteen years. Five major U.S. hospitals now treat with proton therapy, and about 16 more proton facilities are in the design or construction stages. The U.S. FDA has approved its use for treating cancer and other diseases. More than 50,000 patients have been treated with proton therapy. Does this sound like a treatment modality that is *experimental* or *investigational?*

Look at the data and talk with former patients. Proton treatment is non-invasive, painless, and results in fewer side effects. Any objective person will conclude that proton therapy is, in fact, superior to the other forms of treatment.

Appeal and You Will Most Likely Win

One of the BOB's many services is to counsel men who have been denied medical insurance coverage. The first thing we encourage the patient to do is to file an appeal. It is surprising how many companies will reverse their decision on a simple appeal.

If the first appeal doesn't work, we encourage a second appeal, and a third, if necessary. We generally provide the patient/BOB member information and guidance that often works in the appeal process such as:

- Suggesting their physician provide a referral to a proton treatment center.
- The names of patients whose treatment was covered by the very same insurance company that denied their coverage.
- Published research material and data proving the efficacy and superiority of proton therapy.
- Information about Medicare (Bulletin 406, 3/31/97) and Blue Shield of California (Policy 4.01.04, 2/27/97) declaring proton-beam radiation therapy as "non-investigational."
- A statement from the Blue Shield Policy indicates: "Treatment with proton-beam radiation therapy should consider the characteristic absorption in a specified target volume and location that would likely result in superior clinical outcomes as compared to conventional (photons) or electron-beam radiotherapy."
- Patient advocate websites that guide patients through the appeal process (Example: http://www.patientadvocate.org).
- The names of competent attorneys who specialize in insurance appeals. One of the best is Michael Bidart of Shernoff, Bidart,

Darras & Dillon, Claremont, CA. Firms like this one often make claims that denying proton beam coverage is a "fraudulent unfair business practice."

- Statements like the following: How can this treatment be experimental or investigational if more than 50,000 patients have been treated with protons since the early 1950s, and new proton treatment facilities are springing up all over the country (Massachusetts, Indiana, Texas, Florida, Pennsylvania, Virginia, Illinois, Washington, Oklahoma), and in other parts of the world (Australia, Asia, Europe)?
- Copies of successful appeal letters written by our members.

Switch Companies

Another strategy that has worked for many was to switch from their HMO to a PPO or another offering within their own insurance company network. Sometimes this needs to be done during the open enrollment period. Surprisingly, this has been a very successful approach for many. It may take several days or even a few weeks, but it could mean the difference between proton treatment and surgery, or between funding the treatment out of pocket or receiving reimbursement. Since prostate cancer tends to be slow growing, a few weeks of work to switch insurers shouldn't matter.

This approach has worked well for several of our members. When Kaiser Permanente refused to pay for proton therapy, one of our members switched to AARP which, in turn, covered all costs, even though the individual had a preexisting condition. Since that time, several of our members have switched to AARP for insurance coverage when their insurer refused to pay. AARP seems to consistently take the "high road" when it comes to supporting its customers.

Winston Churchill Said It Best

The message here is not to accept the insurance company's denial of coverage. "There are many ways to skin a cat," and there are many ways to secure coverage for this life saving treatment.

Quoting Winston Churchill, "Never, never, never, never, never give up!"

The Preemptive Approach

If you have rising PSA, or are at higher risk for prostate cancer, you may want to check to see if your current insurance carrier reimburses for proton treatment. If not, now is the time to switch to a reputable company that recognizes the value of this treatment and reimburses for it. I have heard numerous stories of HMOs denying coverage for various medical procedures, which suggests that switching out of your HMO may make sense, even if none of the above applies to you *at this time*.

The appendix includes a partial list of medical insurance companies which have been known to reimburse for proton therapy.

CHAPTER 15

What if My Treatment Fails?

"If we don't change, we don't grow. If we don't grow, we are not really living. Growth demands a temporary surrender of security."

-- Gail Sheehy

All is Not Lost

To properly deal with this subject one must first understand what the term "treatment failure" means. Before PSA was used as a relative prostate cancer marker, failure was determined by either prostate cancer symptoms (blood in the urine, pelvic pain, urinary tract problems, etc.) or by the presence of a lump in the prostate area detected by digital rectal exam. As mentioned in an earlier chapter, the term cNED (no Clinical Evidence of Disease) is used to describe this process.

Today, the PSA measurement has added a new dimension to monitoring a patient following prostate cancer treatment, regardless of the treatment chosen. The term bNED (no Biochemical Evidence of Disease) refers to post treatment PSA behaving in a certain fashion.

PSA comes from only two sources: 1) a functioning prostate, or 2) prostate cancer. Therefore, if one chooses surgery and has the prostate removed, post treatment PSA should be non-detectable. Any measurable PSA would indicate the presence of prostate cancer.

For all other treatments, which leave the prostate in place – albeit "damaged" by the treatment process – one would expect to see low levels of PSA in the bloodstream. If the cancer has been destroyed, however, this PSA level, produced by the remaining prostate tissue, and referred to as the *nadir*, should be relatively steady. Multiple increases in PSA following external beam radiation therapy, brachytherapy, or cryosurgery, would be indicative of biochemical failure, thus cancer activity. A single high reading should be no cause for alarm. PSA 'bumps' are common after non-surgical treatments.

If there are multiple PSA increases, indicating the probability of cancer activity (biochemical failure), or if there is clinical failure as detected either by DRE or the presence of prostate cancer symptoms, all is not necessarily lost. This is *not* a death sentence.

PSA Velocity

It is entirely possible, and even likely, that the primary treatment destroyed (or removed) most, but not all of the cancer. The remaining cancer cells, which will produce some PSA in the blood, may continue growing at a rate that is slow enough to be of no concern. This is especially true if the patient is elderly and is likely to die of other causes before the prostate cancer can begin to produce symptoms.

Dr. Charles E. "Snuffy" Myers, Professor of Medicine and Urology, University of Virginia School of Medicine, wrote an excellent article on this subject, referencing studies by R.S. Pruthi and C.R. Pound, both listed in the bibliography in the appendix.

First Steps

In the event the recurrent cancer is growing fast and action is needed, there are several steps that should be taken before any decision could be made on treatment. This could be the subject for another book, but will be summarized here.

The first step might be to determine if the cancer has metastasized to distant parts of the body. If so, there are certain treatments available.

If no metastasis, then the location of the cancer should be determined. A biopsy of the prostate would show if the cancer is there. Other tests, such as ProstaScint and PET Scan could help determine where the recurrent cancer might be located.

Depending on the results of these tests, any one of several salvage treatment options could be prescribed.

Salvage Options

Patients who have undergone any form of external beam radiation therapy have several salvage options available to them if tests show the cancer is still localized within the prostate. These include internal radiation (brachytherapy), cryosurgery, and salvage radical prostatectomy. The latter is more complicated than primary radical prostatectomy, but is being done by specialists in major cancer treatment centers.

High Intensity Focused Ultrasound (HIFU) may also be an alternative, but this procedure is quite new and is not practiced in the United States as of this writing.

When the cancer is determined to be *outside* the prostate, treatment options are more limited. The most common approach is hormone ablation therapy.

Patients who have undergone surgery as their initial treatment have the option of all forms of external beam radiation, as well as hormone therapy, for their salvage treatment.

Numerous vaccines and other treatments are in clinical trials, and the technology is changing almost daily. New primary and salvage treatment options are on the horizon and will undoubtedly be available in the years to come.

Just as in the case of primary treatments, these salvage treatments carry the risk of certain side effects such as impotence, incontinence, and rectal or urinary tract damage.

CHAPTER 16

Ten Steps for Taking Control of The Detection and Treatment of Your Prostate Cancer

"The difference between a successful person and others is not a lack of strength, not a lack of knowledge, but rather in a lack of will."

-- *Vincent Lombardi*

Take Control with these Ten Steps

If you follow these 10 steps, you will greatly increase your chances of catching the disease early. And the earlier this disease is detected, the easier it is to cure.

Equally as important, once diagnosed, there are many things you can do which will virtually guarantee that you make the treatment decision that will give you the best chance of a cure and, most likely, with minimal to no side effects.

1. **Choose your doctors wisely**

2. **Monitor your PSA**

3. **Have an annual DRE**

4. **Have a *Free*-PSA test done**

5. **Manage your biopsy test**

6. **Evaluate all treatment options**

7. **Talk with men who have been through it**

8. **Make your decision based on what is best for you**

9. **Choose the best practitioner and hospital**

10. **Maintain your physical and mental health**

1. Choose Your Doctors Wisely

Primary Care Physician.   This is your first line of defense. Almost all prostate cancers are discovered as a result of action by the patient's family doctor. Too often the cancer is discovered after it has progressed well beyond the early stage, because the patient's doctor was not knowledgeable or didn't recognize the early signs of prostate cancer.

Many people choose the doctor who is closest to their home or office. Others move into a new neighborhood and make their choice based on a neighbor's recommendation. That may be a good start, but you should then meet with the doctor and conduct an interview to ensure that he or she is best for you.

My current primary care physician's office is an hour and a half drive from my home. There are literally hundreds of doctors closer to where I live. I chose this particular physician for the following reasons:

- He is bright and personable.
- He spends time with his patients, carefully and thoughtfully answering all their questions. You are never rushed through an annual physical or an office visit.
- He returns telephone calls within a reasonable time period.
- His specialty is gastroenterology, which is important to me, as both my parents had colon cancer, and this is another disease where heredity and early detection are important factors.

- He has performed hundreds of colonoscopies, the most important early detection test for colon cancer.
- He understands the early signs of prostate cancer and is responsive to rising PSA.
- He keeps abreast of new developments in medicine.
- He is "proton friendly" and has recommended proton therapy to his patients.
- He came highly recommended by a doctor friend, whose opinion I value.

To me, it is worth the long drive to have the best medical care. If there were an emergency, I would go to my local hospital emergency room. For everything else, I make the 1½ hour drive.

The principal function of your primary care physician should be *health protection* and *proactive disease prevention*. Good doctors will not wait for the telltale symptoms of a medical disorder to show up. They will use all the information available to them – physical examinations, routine medical tests, and discussions with their patients – to probe for the earliest sign of an abnormality.

Your automobile engine will run longer and smoother if you ensure the crankcase oil is clean and filled to the proper level and if you take other appropriate preventive maintenance measures. Waiting for the engine to "send you a signal" that something is wrong might be too late; the damage may already be done – and it may be irreversible.

Know your doctor's *opinion* of the PSA test. Many physicians believe that because PSA is a non-specific test for prostate cancer, a high or rising number is not cause for alarm. Or, they may feel PSA is of no concern until it progresses beyond the "normal" range. In both cases there may not be cause for *alarm*, but there *is* cause for *concern* and *action*. This is discussed in the next steps.

Most of us do not see a urologist until a problem is detected or suspected. So your family doctor or primary care physician is your first line of defense against prostate cancer. Choose him or her wisely.

Urologist. Sooner or later just about everyone, male or female, will need a urologist. Why wait until a problem develops? Why not do some homework and select your urologist before there is a medical need? He might not be taking new patients when you need him the most. The best time to select a good urologist is when you don't need one.

Most general practitioners are affiliated with a specific urologist and will typically refer their patients to this associate. That particular urologist may or may not be the best one for you.

If you have prostate cancer in your family, or if you have rising PSA, you should begin the search for a urologist at the earliest opportunity. Find out what doctors your friends and acquaintances use. Check their credentials. What hospital are they affiliated with? What is the reputation of that hospital? What technique do they use to take biopsy samples? How many biopsy core samples do they take? It should be a minimum of 12, preferably 20. Is a local anesthetic used during biopsy sampling?

Speak with patients who use the urologist you are considering. Especially speak with patients who have had prostate biopsies done by this doctor.

Find out if the doctor uses an assistant while taking biopsy samples. This is essential if you want the procedure to be done quickly, efficiently, and with the least amount of discomfort.

Ask how many prostatectomies (surgeries) has he/she done? Find out if this doctor ever recommends anything other than surgery for prostate cancer patients who are younger than 65. Most urologists will suggest other treatment alternatives or watchful waiting for older patients who cannot tolerate the trauma of surgery, so the question is important: Does he/she ever recommend radiation, seeds, cryo, etc. to patients who are younger than 65?

Speak with patients who have had a radical prostatectomy by this doctor. What has been their experience? What were their short and long term side effects? Do they have measurable PSA? Are they considered "cured?" If the surgery failed and the cancer recurred, what follow up treatment did the doctor recommend?

You may not be able to find answers to all these questions, but find out as much as you can.

One service the Brotherhood of the Balloon provides its members is a list of "proton friendly" urologists within the U.S. These are doctors who have treated BOB members and are considered to be excellent physicians with open minds on proton therapy.

2. Monitor Your PSA

This sounds pretty obvious. But it is surprising how many men are not paying attention to their PSA. Either they are not having annual physicals, or their doctor hasn't chosen to have the simple and inexpensive blood test run to measure PSA. I receive calls all the time from men with advanced prostate cancer who fit into one of these two categories.

A 54-year-old highly successful business owner called me with the following story: His last physical was in 1997. At that time he had a PSA of 2.4 and normal DRE. His next physical was six years later, in 2003, at which time his PSA was 60, a DRE revealed a hard mass and all six biopsy samples tested positive for adenocarcinoma, Gleason score 8. By not having routine physicals and monitoring PSA, this man put himself in an extremely vulnerable position with few options and high risk of metastasis, for which there is no cure.

A survey conducted by NOP Healthcare with 1,400 men in the US, UK, France, Germany, Italy, Spain and Sweden showed one-third of men are not familiar with available tests to diagnose prostate cancer.

The most important thing to remember about prostate cancer is that it is curable *if detected early*. Make sure you have a PSA test at least once a year. Most doctors will begin measuring their male patient's PSA at age 50, since prostate cancer is generally not found in men until after that age. My recommendation is to begin at age 45. And, if there is prostate cancer in your family, begin measuring your PSA level at age 40 or sooner. It is wise to have an early "baseline" PSA, especially if you are at higher risk. The test is simple and inexpensive.

If your PSA rises by more than 0.5 ng/ml in one year, consider repeating the test in three months to see if this trend is continuing or possibly accelerating. If the PSA rise exceeds 0.75 in one year, repeat the test in one month. If the retest confirms the 0.75 rise, this is a red flag. Your doctor may want to put you on an antibiotic, such as Cipro, for one month to rule out an infection (prostatitis) as a possible cause. If your PSA continues at that level, or moves higher, talk with your urologist about scheduling a biopsy – *even if your PSA is within the normal range.*

Example: Say that your PSA was 1.5 last year. This year it measures 2.3 (i.e. a greater than 0.75 rise). You retest one month later and the 2.3 is confirmed. Your doctor prescribes Cipro for one month in order to rule out infection as the cause. Retesting one month later confirms the 2.3 reading. Schedule a biopsy – even though your PSA is still within the "normal" range of 0 - 4.

Do not rely solely on your doctor to raise a red flag on this important measurement. You need to monitor your own PSA velocity. Too often, doctors are not alarmed until your PSA level approaches or exceeds the upper limit of the "normal" range (0 to 4.0). Most labs will automatically flag a number that is higher than 4.0, but they won't tell you if your PSA velocity is dangerously high.

Here is a note I received from one of our BOB members who happens to have chosen an excellent family doctor:

"I have been tracking my PSA for ten years. It started at 1.0 and was slowly going up each year. Last year it jumped from 1.9 to 2.4. A repeat PSA test two months before I went to Loma Linda was 2.7. My family doctor, who was giving me my annual physical, not a urologist, knew my family history. My father had passed due to prostate cancer. My mother passed due to breast cancer. He thought that it would be wise for me to get an ultrasound test. He said he had seen other patients who had aggressive cancers with a PSA at 2.4. The ultrasound was a little 'suspicious.'

He then took 8 biopsy samples and one was malignant. I now feel really blessed to have caught this cancer as early as we did. Now I hope I can forget about dying from prostate cancer."

PSA is not an absolute indicator of the presence of cancer. A high PSA does not mean you have cancer and a low PSA does not mean that you don't. However, there is a higher probability that you *have* prostate cancer with higher PSA than with low. Equally important is the fact that rapidly rising PSA, *even within the normal range* can indicate abnormal cell activity and possibly be an early warning of cancer. Some doctors will call attention to this change in PSA within the normal range, but many will not. Therefore it is up to

188

you to be vigilant and to closely monitor your own PSA. Again, remember that this disease is curable if you catch it early.

> *Tip: Keep a file on your PSA measurements. Track them carefully year after year. Plot them on a graph if possible. If a rise of more than 0.75 is observed, even if the number is within the normal range, see your urologist.*

To complicate matters further, recent studies reported in the Journal of Urology have shown that 24.5% of men with PSAs in the upper end (2.5 to 4.0) of the normal range do in fact, have early stage prostate cancer. For this reason we can expect the top of the "normal" PSA range to be adjusted downward sometime in the future.

There is another important reason for finding the cancer at this early stage: It has been amply demonstrated that *cure rates* for patients having prostate cancer with pretreatment PSAs below 4.0 are better than those with pretreatment PSAs above 4.0, regardless of the treatment option chosen.

Don't Panic at a Single High Reading

There can be several reasons for an abnormally high PSA reading. They include:
- Prostate Infection
- BPH a benign condition
- Laboratory error
- Any stimulation of the prostate gland

An article in the August 1998 Journal of Laboratory Medicine quantified some of the non-cancer causes for elevated PSA.

Condition/Manipulation	Effect on PSA Increase	Persists
Acute bacterial prostatitis	5-7 fold	6 weeks
Acute urinary retention	5-7 fold	6 weeks
Exercise - bicycle	0-3 fold	1 week
Prostate biopsy	Very Variable	6 weeks
Prostate massage	Variable	6 weeks
Ejaculation	Variable	3 days
TURP (transurethral resection of the prostate)	Very Variable	6 weeks

A different study added the Digital Rectal Exam to the above list. A DRE performed within 72 hours of drawing blood for PSA can cause elevated readings. Many physicians do not know this: blood should *always* be drawn before the DRE is performed. Stimulation of the prostate by DRE can cause PSA to be elevated.

The bottom line is that any activity that might stimulate the prostate gland should be avoided for several days before a PSA blood test is conducted. Many doctors are surprisingly unaware of this fact, or otherwise fail to communicate this information to their patients. I have spoken with numerous men who reported their doctors typically do the digital rectal examination (DRE) just *before* blood is drawn for the PSA test. Many of these men reported erroneously high readings when the test results come in.

Men often suffer needless anxiety for the several days it takes for the repeat blood test and PSA measurement, only to find out that the elevated reading was a false alarm.

Laboratory mistakes are not uncommon. PSA tests, although somewhat automated, are conducted by human beings, and we humans make mistakes. Despite the best of intentions, occasional errors occur, and they result in false readings.

Tip: At the first sign of an abnormal PSA reading, repeat the test. And, make sure you abstain from any activity that might stimulate the prostate gland for at least three days before the repeat blood test.

Even if a repeat test confirms the higher reading, it is still not necessarily cause for alarm. There are several non-cancer possibilities that need to be ruled out before proceeding to the biopsy step.

Many men have suffered and died from prostate cancer because their doctor did not measure their PSA, or he/she measured it, but didn't pay attention to the results.

It is impossible to track your PSA if your doctor is not submitting blood samples to a laboratory. Also, I have learned that not all doctors do a PSA test during the annual physical examination. Make sure your doctor does.

3. Have an Annual Digital Rectal Exam (DRE)

Why is this so important? Because we cannot rely on PSA alone to send us a signal that a cancer is growing in our prostate. PSA is only a *relative* indicator of prostate cancer. Approximately one out of seven men diagnosed with prostate cancer has a PSA in the normal range. Many more men with "normal" PSAs have undiagnosed prostate cancer. Studies have also shown that one out of four men whose PSA is in the top half of the "normal" range has prostate cancer.

Often, prostate cancer can be detected by the simple Digital Rectal Exam (DRE) test, which literally takes only seconds in the doctor's office. Details of the DRE are discussed in previous chapters. Compared to the horrors of prostate cancer this simple test is a "piece of cake." Yet many men avoid it because it makes them uncomfortable.

Although it is possible to have prostate cancer with normal DRE and PSA in the 0 to 4.0 range, it is likely that one of these two measurements will signal the presence of prostate cancer if it is there.

And remember, *any activity that might stimulate the prostate gland should be avoided for several days before blood is drawn for PSA test.* This includes the DRE.

4. Have a *Free*-PSA Test Done

This is a little used, yet reasonably accurate predictor of prostate cancer. *Free*-PSA should be used when there is suspicion of prostate cancer before a biopsy is ordered. This test could be used to eliminate unnecessary, expensive, and uncomfortable biopsies, according to a survey conducted by the *Men's Health Network.* "The survey suggests many doctors are not yet taking advantage of the risk-assessment information that the *free*-PSA test provides about how likely prostatic biopsies are to show cancers in individual cases," said prostate cancer specialist William J. Catalona, M.D. of the Washington University School of Medicine. "That means patients may not have all the information they need to make an informed decision about whether or not to have a biopsy."

Tip: If your PSA is rising, whether or not it is outside the normal range, consider having a Free-PSA test done in order to predict the likelihood of a positive biopsy. It might help you avoid the cost and discomfort of a needle biopsy.

Free-PSA (FPSA) numbers are expressed in percentages. The higher the percentage, the lower the probability one has prostate cancer. If FPSA is higher than 25% the likelihood of prostate cancer is less than 8%. If FPSA is below 10% the likelihood of cancer is greater than 50%.

The following table shows how PSA and FPSA relate to the probability of one's having prostate cancer. As you can see, when both are used together, the predictability improves. In my case, I had a PSA of 7.9, which indicated a 25% probability. A FPSA of 7% predicted a better than 56% chance of my having prostate cancer. You may recall that I had already had two previous biopsies with negative results. I was not anxious to have a third. However, when the FPSA results came in, I agreed to the biopsy, which ultimately proved to be positive.

PSA	Probability of Cancer
0-2 ng/ml	1%
2-4	15
4-10	25
>10	>50

%FPSA	Probability of Cancer
0-10	56
10-15	28
15-20	20
20-25	16
>25	8

The original of this was presented in the JAMA 279:1543, 1998
*Recent studies show that with PSA levels between **2.5 ng/mL and 4.0 ng/mL** (the current cutoff for prostate cancer screening), cancer was detected on biopsy in **24.5%** of the men, with **67.6%** of cancers being clinically significant. J Urol 2001;165:757-760.*

5. Manage Your Biopsy Test

This important and marginally invasive procedure involves imaging the prostate using a rectally inserted ultrasound tube, and then inserting a device in the rectum that contains a spring-loaded hollow needle to take the sample. The ultrasound helps the doctor position the needle. When the needle is properly positioned, the doctor "pulls the trigger," and the hollow needle passes through the rectal wall and into the prostate gland where it removes a core sample of tissue.

Because this is a sampling technique, the more samples taken, the better your chances of finding the cancer early. Insist on a minimum of twelve biopsy samples, preferably more – my recommendation is 20 samples, 10 in each lobe. A study by Robert Bahnson, Chief of Urology at Ohio State University, indicated that one in seven prostate cancers are missed with a six-sample biopsy.

These would likely be found by doubling the number of samples taken according to the study.

I truly believe that in my case, had I insisted on 20 samples the first time, my cancer would have been diagnosed two years sooner, and I would have been spared two additional biopsy tests. Progressive urologists routinely remove 12, 16, or 20 biopsy samples.

If the cancer is microscopic in size, it can easily be missed by a biopsy needle that removes only six small tissue samples. These few samples represent only a tiny fraction of your prostate's volume. None of us ever want to hear those awful words "you have cancer," but if it *is* going to happen, it is unquestionably in your best interest to *find it early*. Early detection is critically important and will greatly influence the likelihood of a cure. In other words, *proper sampling and early diagnosis can represent the difference between life and death.* At the very least, early diagnosis can have significant impact on the *quality of life* following treatment, as early treatment options tend to be much 'kinder and gentler' than those used for advanced cancers.

> ***Tip: Insist on a minimum of 12 biopsy samples – ideally 20 – to insure the cancer is found at the earliest possible stage.***

There is an additional benefit to taking a larger number of biopsy samples. If the results come back negative, you can have a greater degree of confidence that there really *is* no cancer. In my case, being an engineer familiar with the statistical inaccuracies associated with inadequate sampling, I suspected the cancer was there, even though the first two biopsy reports were negative. I did not know at the time, however, that I could have requested, or rather *insisted*, on 12, 16, or 20 samples. As a result, I gave the cancer an additional two years to grow inside my body, and possibly even migrate to places outside the prostate. I wish *this* book had been available to me back then!

One additional point (no pun intended) on needle biopsies. They do not have to be painful. Some urologists offer a local anesthesia to patients to make them more comfortable during the procedure. This takes a little more time, but it is well worth it. A Lidocaine injection or nitrous oxide (laughing gas), for example, can significantly reduce pain during a prostate biopsy. If your urologist doesn't offer the option of pain management for the biopsy test –

especially for a 20 sample biopsy – I would recommend finding a new urologist.

6. Evaluate All Treatment Options

If you are diagnosed with prostate cancer do not rely on the first recommendation made by your urologist. Unless you are too old or too weak to handle the trauma, he/she will most likely recommend surgery. Remember, urologists are surgeons, and for years, the "gold standard" for prostate cancer treatment has been surgery. Some of us have come to believe that surgery should be called "the *old* standard." There are non-invasive treatment options that offer comparable cure rates without the trauma, blood loss, side effects, or recovery time of surgery.

Tip: Examine all the treatment options and choose the right one for you. Do not let your physician make that decision for you.

Learn about the male anatomy, the location and function of the prostate. Learn everything you can about each of the treatment options you are considering.

If you are considering a radical prostatectomy, learn how the procedure is done. Evaluate all other non-invasive options before choosing surgery. Remember *you* are the one on the receiving end of the scalpel.

If your cancer stage is anything other than early stage, consider having a bone scan, whether or not your doctor recommends it. This important test will help determine if the cancer has metastasized, i.e. traveled to distant parts of your body. Once you have ruled out metastasis, your options are many. Proton treatment was best for me. It may not be for you. Others have been successfully treated by the other options listed in earlier chapters.

Put together your own decision matrix. Assign the most weight to those factors which are most important to you. Perhaps taking two months out of your life to be away from family and work is absolutely out of the question. This would rule out proton treatment – unless you live near one of the treatment centers and can continue your normal work routine while in treatment.

Perhaps the minimal hospital stay of brachytherapy, combined with quick recovery is most important to you, even if certain side effects have a higher probability of occurring. Or, perhaps you may feel strongly about having the gland with the cancer removed from your body as soon as possible, and thus prefer the oldest method, surgery.

7. Talk With Men Who Have Been Through It

Prostate cancer is slow growing. It took years for it to grow to the point where it was detected in your body. You do not have to make the decision today, this week, or even this month. Take the time to do your research. Buy and read the best books on the subject. Research the Internet. And, above all, *talk with several men who have had each of the treatments you are considering.*

Remember, most books on this subject are written by doctors or researchers who haven't been through the treatment. Only someone who has been through it can truly relate to you their personal experience. Make up your own list of questions for these former patients representing each treatment option.

Include questions such as these:

Why did you choose surgery (or brachytherapy, or external beam radiation etc.)? Did you do extensive research? Or, did you just accept your urologist's recommendation?

Did you consider any other treatment option? If so, why did you disregard them?

What was your experience of this treatment? Was it positive? Was there a lot of pain, blood loss, or complications?

What short term side effects did you experience? How long did they last?

What long-term side effects have you experienced?

Ask specific questions about incontinence. Did you experience any incontinence – bladder control problems? Do you have any leakage today? If so, under what conditions?

Ask specific questions about impotence. Have you experienced any changes in sexual function? Are erections the same today as they were before treatment?

When did you have this procedure done? What was your pretreatment PSA, Gleason score, and T-score? What is your PSA today? (Remember, if he had surgery, and the prostate was removed, his PSA should be non-detectable. If he had any other procedure, he still has a prostate, so there should be a low level of measurable PSA, and it should be dropping or holding steady, if he has reached nadir.)

Would you choose this procedure again? This will tell you a lot about this patient's overall evaluation of the option he chose. Several of the men I talked with told me they felt they made the wrong choice.

What advice do you have for me? We can always learn from another patient's experience. If he chose the same treatment option you are considering, perhaps he can tell you about ways to prepare for your treatment or give you ideas that will make your experience less anxiety filled and even enjoyable. I received numerous helpful suggestions and recommendations from former proton patients.

Can you give me the names and phone numbers of others who have had prostate cancer treatment? *You can never talk with too many former patients.* You will learn more from them than from the doctors, the books, or the Internet, *especially if you question them in depth.*

8. Make Your Decision Based on What Is Best For You

Involve your wife (or significant other), your loved ones, and even your closest friends in the decision. Perhaps they will think of something you have not considered. Either way, their involvement in your decision will solidify your thinking and commitment to the option you choose. Their involvement will also help erase any doubts you might have as to whether your choice is the best option for you.

If you follow a spiritual path, pray about the decision. For me this was a most important factor. The more I prayed, the more confident I became that proton treatment was best for me.

9. Choose the Best Practitioner and Hospital

One gentleman from Canada told me he was considering brachytherapy with a local physician. I asked him how many his doctor had performed. He told me he'd check. When he called back, he told me, "She's done six." I said, "Six per day or per week?" He said, "No, six in total." My response was, "Why not let her practice on someone else?"

There are significant variations in the results being seen by different doctors and hospitals around the world, both in terms of cure rates and side effects for the *same* procedure. You owe it to yourself to find out about these differences and to pick a doctor and hospital that has demonstrated the best results. If this means traveling a long distance, then so be it. What is the price of maintaining your potency or bladder control? Certainly the inconvenience or additional cost of some travel should be worth the benefit.

10. Maintain Your Physical and Mental Health

Regardless of the option you choose, your physical and mental health, as well as your attitude can make a huge difference in the overall experience and outcome of your treatment. Studies have shown those in better physical health and those with a positive mental attitude statistically have quicker recoveries and higher cure rates.

Perhaps this is because the body's immune system is an important factor in preventing the growth and spread of cancer. Better physical and mental health supports a stronger immune system.

If not already actively involved in a physical fitness program, begin now. This can be as simple as walking a mile or two a day. Otherwise join a fitness club and work out three or four times a week. Include exercise that would improve cardiovascular fitness, such as jogging, stationary bike, rowing machine, or stair climber. Of course you should check with your doctor before engaging in any new physical activity.

Eat a healthy diet. This means minimizing red meats, processed meats, animal fats, and most dairy products. Introduce healthy foods into your diet, such as soy products, fresh fruits, and vegetables. Exercise regularly and maintain proper body weight. Take vitamins and supplements to supply your body with nutrients missing from your diet. All these things can both slow, or stop, the progress of prostate cancer and help prevent a recurrence.

If you are in a high risk group (family history, African American) be extra vigilant with regard to diet, exercise, and monitoring the key measurements.

If you have significant anxiety about your diagnosis and your decision, speak with your priest, minister, or rabbi. Talk with your doctor or a therapist. Perhaps short term anti-depressant or anti-anxiety medication would help you through the "rough spots."

Frequent communications with men who have been successfully treated for prostate cancer can be of great benefit. There are Internet chat rooms, newsletters, man-to-man organizations and support groups of all types available to you. Joining a support group can do much to improve your knowledge, your attitude, and your confidence in the outcome of your treatment for prostate cancer.

Summary

Someone once asked me, "What do you call the guy who graduated at the bottom of his class in medical school?" I said, "I don't know; what do they call him?" The answer, "Doctor."

Not all doctors are created equally. Even some very intelligent doctors are one-dimensional. They may have great diagnostic skills in certain areas of medicine, and be quite uninformed in others. Many diseases and health disorders have obvious telltale signs that any doctor can easily identify. Prostate cancer is *not* one of them.

The best doctors may not be located in your community. You owe it to yourself to choose the best family doctor and urologist you can find, even if it means traveling some distance to see them.

Monitoring your own PSA and having an annual DRE will greatly increase your chances of finding the cancer at an early – and thus treatable – stage. The combination of these measurements actually gives you three tools:

1. **Absolute PSA number**. The top half of the range (2 – 4) is a caution sign. A reading over 4.0 is a red flag.
2. **A rise in PSA** of 0.75 or greater in one year is also a red flag, even if it is within the normal range.
3. **The presence of a lump**, hardness, or other abnormality by DRE is another warning signal.

A prostate biopsy should be done if:

A. Your PSA is over 4.0, you have ruled out infection as the cause, and a Free PSA test indicates the probability of cancer.
B. Your PSA is in the 2 to 4 range, you have family history of prostate cancer, and Free PSA suggests the probability of cancer.
C. Your PSA rises 0.75 units or more in one year (even within the normal range) and you have ruled out lab error or infection.
D. The DRE test detects a lump or hardness in the prostate (regardless of whether PSA is rising or is elevated).

Insist on a minimum twelve-sample biopsy, preferably twenty-sample, ten in each lobe. With early stage prostate cancer, the more samples, the easier it is to find.

Ask your doctor for local anesthesia to eliminate the discomfort of the test. He or she can't feel it, why should you?

If you are diagnosed with prostate cancer, educate yourself on all treatment options. Several books are referenced in the appendix. Explore the Internet. Attend support group meetings in your community. Above all, *interview prostate cancer patients who have completed the treatments you are considering.*

Choose the best option for *you*. This choice should include the best (or one of the top five) doctors and hospitals practicing this treatment option. If you decide on brachytherapy (seed implant) for example, and select a local radiation oncologist to do the procedure because it's *convenient*, you may be doing yourself a great disservice. Seed implant is extremely practitioner dependent. If you cannot have the procedure done by one of the best doctors in the field, choose another treatment option.

Finally, remember that your immune system plays an important role in your body's ability to fight off the growth or spread of cancer, before and after treatment. Give your immune system every possible chance to do its job. Eat a healthy diet; make selective vitamins and supplements a part of your daily routine; and take positive steps to maintain or improve your physical and mental health.

Prostate cancer is a serious disease, but it does not have to be a death sentence. The earlier it is caught, the better your chance of beating it. With the information presented in this book, there is no reason why you should have to die of prostate cancer, or have the quality of your life significantly impacted by the treatment option you choose.

Remember, the most common symptom of prostate cancer is *no symptom at all*. Don't wait for a symptom to appear. If you do, it may be too late.

If you follow the advice given in this book, you will undoubtedly die some day – but it will likely not be from prostate cancer.

Final Thought

The thought I would like to leave you with is this: Prostate cancer is not a death sentence. If you properly educate yourself, *you* can take control of *your* diagnosis and treatment. For me this has been a most incredible journey, one I wouldn't swap for anything in the world.

Remember: *You can beat prostate cancer, and you don't need surgery to do it.*

I wish you good luck and good health, and I welcome your e-mails at RMarckini@protonbob.com, with comments, questions and suggestions.

APPENDIX

Appendix A

Terms and Abbreviations

Adenocarcinoma	This is the most common cancer of the prostate. It begins in the glandular cells that produce prostatic fluid.
Biopsy	This procedure involves the removal of multiple tissue samples from the prostate using a spring-loaded needle. Six to twenty samples are typically taken. Local anesthesia is recommended to minimize discomfort. Some blood is often found in the urine and semen for days or weeks following a prostate biopsy.
Bone Scan	Bone Scan is a 2-Dimensional image of the skeleton using a radioactive tracer. This is a common test to detect cancer that has spread to the bone, a favorite site for prostate cancer to go to.
BPH	Benign Prostatic Hyperplasia. A non-cancerous condition of the prostate gland. It typically refers to an enlarged prostate which may cause a pinching of the urethra and restriction of urine flow. This is a common condition in older men.
Brachytherapy	Seed Implant therapy. 80 to 120 radioactive seeds are implanted in the prostate, destroying cancer by radiating the gland from within.
Chest X-Ray	Chest X-Ray (CXR) is a 2-Dimensional image of the lung, ribs, and back bone using x-rays. A CXR is commonly used to detect the spread of cancer to the chest area and for screening for other diseases.
Cryosurgery	Extremely low temperature liquid nitrogen freezing of the prostate and tumor.
CT Scan	Computerized Tomography (CT) is a 3-Dimensional image of the body using x-rays. CT

	is a commonly used 3-D imaging tool to help detect cancer that has metastasized (spread) beyond the tissue or organ where it started from. CT is useful when looking for the spread of cancer into the nearby bone and lymph nodes.
DRE	Digital Rectal Examination. A gloved finger in inserted into the rectum in order to feel the prostate gland to determine if there are any abnormalities.
EBRT	External Beam Radiation Therapy, generally thought to be photon, or X-ray radiotherapy, but it also includes other forms of radiation, including proton.
Free PSA (FPSA)	Refers to the percentage of unbound PSA to bound PSA. The higher the Free PSA percentage, the lower the probability of prostate cancer.
Gleason Score	Refers to the measure of the aggressiveness of the cancer and an indirect predictor of the likelihood the cancer has spread beyond the prostate capsule. Six to twenty tissue samples are taken by needle biopsy and are examined under the microscope. Two areas where cancer is found are graded on a scale of 1 through 5. The two grades are added together to yield the Gleason Score, which ranges from 2 to 10.
HIFU	HIFU (high intensity focused ultrasound) is a procedure that uses high intensity, focused ultrasound to heat and destroy diseased tissue.
Hormone Therapy	Also known as Hormone Ablation Therapy (HAT) or Androgen Deprivation Therapy (ADT). This treatment, often used in conjunction with other therapies is intended to shut down the production of male sex hormones (androgens), such as testosterone.
IMRT	Intensity Modulated Radiation Therapy, an advanced form of X-ray, or photon, external beam radiation therapy.
Morbidity	In the context of evaluating prostate cancer treatment alternatives, the term "morbidity" refers to side effects. These can be further characterized

	as Grade 1, 2 or 3 gastrourinary or gastrointestinal morbidity.
MRI	Magnetic Resonance Imaging (MRI) is a 3-Dimensional image of the body using magnets and radio waves that is very different than a CT. Some of our tissues and organs are seen better by a CT, some by MRI, and some by combining both. MRI is useful to detect the spread of cancer in the soft tissues.
PBT	Proton Beam Therapy or Proton Treatment
PET Scan	Positron Emission Tomography scans use radioactive materials to determine the presence of a tumor. Whole body PET Scans are commonly done to detect cancer.
PIN	Prostatic Intraepithelial Neoplasia. This is a pre-cancerous stage of tissue, observed from prostate biopsy, that may become cancerous in the future. Some pathologists do not consider PIN significant.
ProstaScint	Uses antibodies attached to radioactive tracers. The antibodies find and attach themselves to the wall of prostate cancer cells. A scan shows "hot spots," which are potential cancer locations.
Prostatitis	A common infection of the prostate.
PSA Test	Prostate Specific Antigen Test, the standard test which may indicate cancer activity in the prostate. The measurement is in nanograms per milliliter, or millionths of grams per thousandth of a liter.
PSA Velocity	The rate at which PSA is rising, usually expressed in terms of "PSA doubling time."
RP	Radical Prostatectomy or surgical removal of the prostate
Staging	This refers to the degree to which the cancer has progressed. There are two staging systems: ABCD and TNM. The TNM is more commonly used today. T represents the prostate cancer stage, expressed as T1, T2, T3, etc. followed by a letter a, b, or c. N represents any involvement of the local lymph nodes. M refers to whether or not there is any distant metastasis.

TRUS	Transrectal Ultrasound. High frequency sound waves are used to determine if there are any abnormalities in the prostate.
TURP	TURP: "transurethral resection of the prostate"... surgery to remove tissue obstructing the urethra. The technique involves inserting an instrument called a resectscope into the urethra, and is intended to relieve obstruction of urine flow due to enlargement of the prostate.
Watchful Waiting or Active Surveillance	Choosing no clinical treatment, generally on the belief that the tumor is slow growing and will not be of harm for the patient's remaining lifespan.

Appendix B

Proton Patient Testimonials

(Examples from our website, www.protonbob.com)

Harold Rabin - Northbrook, Illinois

Treated with Proton therapy in early 1991, Harold Rabin has been cancer free for 15 years, and with no long term side effects.

In 1990 Harold had angioplasty following a heart attack. Two months later he was diagnosed with prostate cancer. His urologist, who favored surgery, expressed some concern about the trauma of a radical prostatectomy. This prompted Harold to begin a search for an alternative treatment. He investigated cryosurgery, which was new at the time, and spoke with his wife's cousin, a medical doctor doing research at the National Institute of Health in Bethesda, MD. The doctor didn't hesitate. He said, "Go to Loma Linda. They are using Protons to kill cancer, and this exciting technology works. Besides, one of my former colleagues at NIH is there now."

Harold visited Loma Linda and was accepted for treatment in early 1991. He remembers telling his urologist about his choice to do Proton therapy at Loma Linda. His mood abruptly changed, according to Harold. "All of a sudden I wasn't 'Harold' anymore, I was 'Mr. Rabin.'" And his next comment was, "Mr. Rabin, if you want to be in an experimental program, that's your business."

Harold commuted from his home in Palm Desert, 110 miles round trip each day for eight weeks - age 70 at the time - and "had the most wonderful experience of my life." He recalls, "Dr. John Antoine was my physician at Loma Linda, and he was terrific. Also, a young physician by the name of Carl Rossi was starting around that time."

When asked about his recollections of Loma Linda 13 years ago, Harold noted that only one gantry was operating. The set-up and treatment took about a half hour. Also, "I left the hospital each day with magic marker marks all over my body." But most of all, he remembers, "the people there were the most pleasant, most wonderful, most gracious, and most professional I have ever met."

It took about four years for Harold's PSA to reach a nadir of 0.3, and there it has stayed for the past eleven years. To say Harold is happy with his results is an understatement. He remembers having a few episodes of rectal bleeding, but "that's been gone for years." And he has experienced no other side effects from his treatment.

I mentioned to Harold that his 1991 treatment date makes him a desirable reference for those considering Proton therapy. I asked if he would consider having his name added to the former patient "Call List" for prospective patients. He said, "Absolutely! I remember how fearful I was when I was diagnosed. And, if people hadn't helped me, I never would have found Loma Linda."

There's something about Proton therapy that attracts the nicest people.

Harold Rabin - Northbrook Illinois
E-mail: hmr111@msn.com

Update added May 1, 2006:

On May 4th 2006 I will be celebrating my 15th year of freedom from Prostate cancer thanks to the wonderful Doctors and staff and the proton treatment I received at Loma Linda. On May 5th I will be celebrating my 85th birthday. What a wonderful birthday present.

I spoke with Harold in October of 2006. He continues to work out regularly in a gym; he plays golf 2 or 3 times a week; and he feels terrific. He promotes proton therapy

---

Robert Hillis, M.D. - Niceville Florida

Dr. Hillis is a surgeon. When diagnosed with prostate cancer, he did his homework and chose proton therapy. On September 19, 2005, The Florida Daily News did a feature story on his diagnosis and treatment at Loma Linda.

"I have a very close friend who was diagnosed with prostate cancer approximately two years ago. He had heard of Loma Linda and proton treatment from a friend, so he chose to go to Loma Linda as well. He told me about his decision and the reasons he had chosen proton treatment. At the time, I had no idea that I would ever be diagnosed with prostate cancer. I had always been very healthy (still am) and there was absolutely no history of prostate cancer in my family. So I listened to my friend and it sounded like he had made a wise decision, but I did no personal research on the subject. After all, I was healthy with no clue I would have the same choice to make in the very near future.

It happened very quickly. In July 2004, I had a routine PSA test, which was returned as 4.9. My urologist said he didn't think I had prostate cancer, but he felt a biopsy was indicated. The DRE was negative and even after the biopsy he felt that the biopsy would come back negative since he didn't see anything with the ultrasound during the biopsy. When I called back a week later, the nurse said the biopsy had been positive - a Gleason of 6.

As most of us are when we hear that horrible word, I was numb and in shock. I'm too healthy to have prostate cancer and no one else in my family has ever had it. When I came back to reality, I asked my urologist what treatment he would have if he were the patient. Surprise! He said he would have surgery. He didn't recommend any other treatment so I told him I would think about it.

I remembered my friends glowing praise of Loma Linda and his treatment. So I went home and got on the Internet and, as a surgeon would do, researched all of my options. I was quite impressed with the medical research regarding proton treatment. After completing my personal research, the decision was a 'no-brainer' for me . . . proton treatment. I called LLUMC and started the process. After sending my medical records, Loma Linda called back saying I was a candidate and an appointment was made. My wife started calling the various housing choices, and since we had an older dog that we wanted to accompany us, we made reservations at Centrepoint.

We were soon on the road and arrived at Loma Linda on Oct 13. They made a final determination that I was a good candidate and my pod was made. Treatments started one week later, and I was back home in Niceville Florida on the 21st of December.

I have some residual symptoms associated with benign prostatic hyperplasia (which I had prior to treatment) and some decrease in endurance, but no other significant post treatment problems. I have had two exams since completion of treatment: DRE's negative and PSA falling. As I said in the newspaper article, Loma Linda was a spiritual awakening event as well as a physical treatment. We enjoyed our time there, traveling around southern California and making lots of friends. Since returning, I have had many inquires from others regarding proton treatment and Loma Linda, and I know of at least one other person who has followed my advice and received treatment at Loma Linda. I continue to recommend Loma Linda to people, as I feel proton is the best treatment and Loma Linda is the best place to receive that treatment."

E-mail: HillisMD@cox.net

Bob Reimer - Arnold, California

"The doctor started off the conversation with "You have cancer and have one to three years to live. Go home and get your affairs in order!"

In December 1997 my internist called, telling me I had a high PSA and he thought I had an infection. After ten days of antibiotics and another PSA he called again and told me to see a urologist ASAP - tomorrow! (Note: I had physicals every year, but was never told my PSA.) I asked the doctor every year, and his answer was always, "Your prostate is slightly enlarged but normal for your age". I told him every year that I wanted to know early, if there was a problem. I have since found out he doesn't believe PSAs mean anything.

After seeing the urologist in January 1998 and having the biopsies done, he waited until February to get the results. The doctor started off the conversation with "You have cancer and have one to three years to live. Go home and get your affairs in order! We were shocked as I felt good and had no symptoms of prostate cancer. I was immediately started on Zolodex, a shot every month.

My wife and I were both in shock but were able to quickly do research and see other doctors. We have a son-in-law who is a doctor and our daughter who is a nurse. They were very helpful with our research.

Since I had a friend who went to Loma Linda for Proton treatment the year before, I made an appointment for an interview. We spent an hour with Dr. Jabola who answered all our questions and was very honest with me. Since my PSA was 61 and Gleason 10+ Dr. Jabola felt I probably would not be a candidate since the cancer was most likely outside the prostate. He had me get a "prostascint" and a scan of the entire torso after taking isotopes four days before. Much to our surprise and joy they found the cancer was still localized.

We immediately let Loma Linda know, and I started Proton in early July 1998. I had fifteen Proton and twenty five photon. The only side effects were diarrhea the last few weeks, and I take a Flomax occasionally if I have trouble urinating. I have seen my PSA go down continually and have no side effects after nearly four and a half years.

We are Christians and have felt God's presence guiding us all the way. The prayers of people, the support of friends and family, and the wonderful care and love shown to us both at Loma Linda are beyond description! God is good. He still heals and gives great peace in times that seem hopeless.

I am available to anyone who has questions or needs a shoulder to cry on.

Bob Reimer - Arnold, California
E-mail: reimer@goldrush.com

Dr. Terry Wepsic – Huntington Beach, CA
(Dr. Wepsic is a noted pathologist and cancer researcher)

Following is part of Dr. Terry Wepsic's Testimonial:

To the Editor of the Wall Street Journal:

"I appreciated your recent article on prostate cancer treatment using Proton Therapy. I am age 63, Yale Medical School Graduate, NIH trained, academic physician/pathologist/ administrator/ educator who has investigated cancer for over thirty years. I have been the primary instructor for second year medical students, introducing them to cancer biology. I was diagnosed with early stage prostate cancer in December 2002, and received proton therapy at Loma Linda University Medical Center. As a sophisticated consumer who is well insured, I could have chosen any form of treatment at any location in the country. I was shocked to reconfirm diagnosis of my own cancer on the lab's pathology slides. Treatment options included laparoscopic surgery at the Henry Ford Hospital in Detroit, brachytherapy at the Seattle Prostate Institute and Proton Beam Therapy at Loma Linda.

Proton beam therapy is totally different from any other form of radiation therapy. Energy from the proton is released only when they stop traveling. Eighty-five to ninety percent of the protons go to the prostate. Only ten percent go to surrounding adjacent tissue. This is in contrast to an effective dose of sixty percent for gamma radiation. Protons can be precisely targeted by exact positioning of the patient and the beam. Radiation can include the area surrounding the prostate capsule and the seminal vesicles. These are two areas where tumor spread can occur, even in early stages of disease. The protons can be tightly focused, and are at present being used to treat wet macular degeneration of the eye in addition to prostate cancer. The macula is about the size of a large grain of rice. Approximately 33,000 patients have been treated worldwide with proton radiation, including cancer of the brain and spinal cord. The cure rate for prostate cancer is comparable to all other forms of treatment, and the side effect profile for erectile dysfunction and incontinence are lower. Many patients have had full post-treatment recovery, including myself.

Loma Linda has led the way with proton therapy for prostate cancer for over fifteen years. Approximately 150-175 prostate cancer patients receive treatment every day, with two shifts being run in four treatment areas. Treatment takes about eight weeks. Patients and their spouses have positive, enjoyable interactions including golf outings, tourist trips and a weekly support group filled with healing humor and concern. Many of these activities are sponsored by the social work staff at Loma Linda. A very supportive web site has been formed at www.protonbob.com. The web site publishes an informative and educational newsletter for over 2000 members.

The best part of my experience was that my primary physician at Loma Linda Medical Center was a former medical student of mine. I have been "beamed up'" as Scotty would say, and I am a better person for this experience. Onward to building more proton centers so treatment advances can occur worldwide."

H. Terry Wepsic, M.D.
Professor Emeritus of Pathology, University of California, Irvine, CA Research Professor at Long Beach V.A. Healthcare System, Long Beach, CA E-mail: capttw@aol.com

---

David Leighton - Foresthill, California

When David Leighton's radical prostatectomy failed, he chose proton treatment to go after the cancer cells the surgery had missed. That was 5 years ago. Today things are looking great!

Proud to be aboard the Brotherhood. This is an outstanding program. I am a solid believer in the "Proton," and your organization is right on track getting the message out to all those in need. Keep up the good work! Early detection and Proton treatment is the way to go!

10-17-95, the prostate biopsy came back hot in the upper left quadrant of the prostate.

12-12-95. my prostate was removed.

214

Two years later, the PSA began to climb again.

11-20-97, ProstaScint - UCLA - indicated cancer in the prostrate bed.
1-26-98, City of Hope, consulted with Dr. Wawachi regarding regular or Proton radiation. PSA 7.

4-98, Started Proton radiation - Proton all the way.

Completed Proton, 2nd week of June 98.

So far, PSA is Non Detectable.

Had no radiation side effects, whatsoever.

That's my history.

Thanks so much, Bob for having me aboard. Looking forward to communicating with all members!

David Leighton - Foresthill, California
E-mail: dglmojo@accessbee.com

Arnd Hallmeyer M.D. - Berlin, Germany

"PSA 436 - good heavens!"

My name is Arnd Hallmeyer. I'm living in Berlin, Germany working as a physician in the field of occupational medicine. I was 57 yrs. when I was diagnosed with prostate cancer. PSA 436 (PSA 436 - good heavens!), Gleason app. 5 (not common in Germany), 4 of 7 biopsy cylinders with adenocarcinoma.

In the beginning of my professional life I worked as a nurse in surgery and after the medical education as a surgeon. I participated in some surgeries of prostate cancer patients, and I still remember all the bad situations of these poor patients as I became older. I never have had any problems or symptoms in relation to urination or sexual things. And, I did not undertake any prostate cancer check-ups. I was afraid of ever being faced with the diagnosis of prostate cancer and having to go through the same terrible experience of radical prostate surgery because I have seen the outcomes of impotence, castration, and wearing diapers for the rest of my life. The decision I made was NOT to contact any urologist. To me, it seemed to be better to die than to live a life after prostate surgery.

Once I developed heavy bone pain, my wife - also a physician and my personal family doctor - started to do several investigations. She was also searching for tumor markers - and of course PSA. The surprising PSA result was   436!

I became deeply depressed, thinking of the end of my life. I remembered my father who tragically died at the age of 58 yrs. from prostate cancer and lots of metastasis in the liver and kidneys.

Now it was my wife's turn and she was to do her job with me as she had done with other patients. She sent my results to one of the best urologists and he started searching for the best hospital and the best surgeon for treating prostate cancer.

When I was asking a well-known radiologist for the best surgeon he knows, his answer was: "You don't need any surgeon, all you need is Loma Linda!" I never heard this name before and had no idea what Loma Linda was. Is this a medicine or a mystic? "No", he answered, "It's the only place in the world you can be healed". That's when I called my daughter Sigrun - also a physician who worked in a large hospital in Harrisburg, Pennsylvania and now in Chicago - and asked her about Loma Linda. She made a lot of phone calls, did Internet research and found a way to Loma Linda University Medical Center, to Prof. James Slater, Dr. Rossi and Sharon Hoyle.

We had some difficulties because of the distance between Loma Linda and Germany and - more - because of the very high PSA. Lian Funada and all the nice women of the department of the International Circle of Care of the LLUMC did a great job and took me into the line.

In the middle of December 2000, I made my first visit to Loma Linda and started the treatment in the early days of January 2001. I received Protons, and - because of the extremely high PSA - photon treatments, too. In addition I received hormone blockers for more safety.

When I came to Loma Linda everything was foreign to me. I didn't have any experience being a patient. I never visited a doctor or a hospital as a patient before in my life. And I didn't have experience with living a daily life in the USA: I had to rent an apartment, a car, and a phone, and I was doing all of the daily work such as shopping, cooking, washing clothes, cleaning the rooms, etc.

My English at that time was very poor and I had some language difficulties, too. But it was very surprising to me, to find lots of good friends suddenly. Each person I met in and around the hospital, in the Proton Treatment Center and in the international circle of care was so friendly and helpful to me. I got the feeling of not being a stranger or patient but coming home to a family after a journey. And for me as a physician and now a patient it was very impressive to experience the benefits of the whole treatment and the care of the employees. The people of the LLUMC were not only treating the disease, they were also healing the bad shape of the soul and sharing the special spirit of Loma Linda. And I found more and more friends: Gerry Troy, Cal Jones and the Wednesday night group, Lynn Martell and the nice people of the office of advancement, and - finally - Bob Marckini and Jerry Klein and the Brotherhood of the Balloon and lots more of unknown names. This way I was able to adapt to the situation. I changed the treatment time to early in the morning or the late evening and got a chance to do outings and to go hiking in the high mountains of the San Bernardino valley several times. Coming closer to heaven, I found a better way back to earth.

I graduated in March 08, 2001 and continued the hormone blockers one more year which included terrible hot flashes and which stopped in January 2002. The last measurement of PSA was undetectable (Sept 2002). I only got negative side effects from the hormone blockers. I experienced no urinary bleedings, no pain, but only some intermittent rectal bleeding in August/September 2002.

Now I'm doing fine overall. I found the road again, and I'm living my life close to normal, back to my daily work. I became a member of the LLUMC International Advisory Council. Together with James Slater, Jerry Slater, Jon Slater and all the good friends of the LLUMC, one of the best private hospitals in Berlin and also good German friends we are on the way to establish a Proton treatment unit in Berlin. It is not simply about making a 1:1 copy of the Loma Linda proton treatment center but to bring the benefits and the spirit of Loma Linda to Europe in order to cure their children, women, and men from cancer in a safe way without pain, hair-loss, hazard or unacceptable side effects.

If you ever get the chance, visit the monument of the Good Samaritan in the yard of Loma Linda University and get a sense of the Loma Linda spirit yourself. Thankfully remembering the days of my second birth in Loma Linda.
Arnd Hallmeyer M.D. - Berlin, Germany
E-mail: ahallmeyer@aol.com

Alex Plummer - Simi Valley, California

"African-Americans, such as Plummer, are 60 percent more likely to develop prostate cancer than Caucasians. "

Reprinted by permission of the *Simi Valley Star*

PROSTATE CANCER SURVIVOR ON A MISSION

By Tim Tanner, Correspondent

July 29, 2002

A routine blood test changed Alex Plummer's life.

It was 1998, and the Simi Valley man was poised to retire from Plummer Security, a company he had run for 20 years. He had big plans, including spending time traveling with his wife, Betty, and the rest of the family.

The blood test, however, showed Plummer had a high level of prostate-specific antigen, an indicator of possible prostate cancer. Plummer, now 69, knew well what the test meant -- his father, Sonny, died at the age of 53 from the disease.

Prostate cancer is the most common form of cancer among men in California. And African-Americans, such as Plummer, are 60 percent more likely to develop prostate cancer than Caucasians.

When Plummer's diagnosis was confirmed, he remembered what his father went through. "I didn't want to be cut or have someone ripping up my body," said Plummer, who now spends his time trying to enlighten men about the options available when prostate cancer is diagnosed.

Plummer said fear and depression set in after his diagnosis. He regularly worked out at a local gym, but began skipping exercise regimens. He closed his security company.

"I use to go to church with my wife, but I turned to the television and watched my favorite preacher, Charles Stanley," Plummer said.

His brother, Miller Plummer, a deacon in a church in New York, called him daily. "God will heal you -- if you have a strong faith and trust in God," Miller told him.

Then Plummer watched a "60 Minutes" segment devoted to proton-beam radiation, a non-surgical alternative to fighting prostate cancer. The procedure was available in Southern California at Loma Linda University Medical Center.

His insurance plan rejected the proton-beam treatments, which cost about $70,000, and said he should have surgery. Plummer said no.

Changing insurance took months, but finally he was allowed to go to Loma Linda and receive 15 proton-beam radiation treatments. Three years later, his cancer remains in remission.

Now, he's determined to stay active and promote prostate cancer awareness. He stresses the importance of men undergoing screening for the disease. Those diagnosed with it should seek opinions from several doctors and then explore various methods of treatment, Plummer said.

A first-person account of his experience appeared in a recent issue of "Guideposts" magazine. And Plummer spreads his prostate cancer message wherever he can -- at support group meetings, at church and in low-income communities of Los Angeles.

"Most people of minority descent have no knowledge of prostate cancer," Plummer said. "I want them to get tested and have a positive attitude. If you start thinking negatively, then it will affect your lifestyle and cause you to deteriorate.

"If you have family support and a positive attitude, you can get through it."

Alex Plummer - Simi Valley, California

Dr. Bernard Hindman (Cambria, CA)

We ran a Featured Member Story on Dr. Bernard Hindman in our BOB Tales Newsletter, and with Dr. Hindman's permission, we posted it on our website as his testimonial. Dr. Hindman is a man of considerable intellect and accomplishment. His story and his rationale for choosing proton therapy should be of great value to recently diagnosed men.

My name is Bernie Hindman and I am a physician. I spent my early life if Florida, where I received a Bachelor of Science degree and Doctor of Medicine, both from the University of Miami. Shortly after graduation from medical school, I married a Florida State University nursing student, Carol Webb, and we have been happily married for 43 years. I am the father of four children, three daughters and a son, and am blessed with twelve grandchildren. My wife and I began our married life in San Francisco, where she was a nurse at Letterman General Hospital. I interned at the Southern Pacific Memorial Hospital, and following the completion of my internship year, I entered the United States Navy as a general medical officer.

After completing my service tour, I returned to the University of Miami, and completed a residency in radiology. My first position was in a suburb of Sacramento, California, where I did general diagnostic radiology. I received my board certification in December, 1970. I practiced in the Sacramento area until 1977, and then following a brief stay in south Florida, I took a Fellowship in pediatric radiology at the Children's Hospital of Los Angeles. After completion of the fellowship, I moved a short distance away to Orthopaedic Hospital, and was there for the next 14 years, the last three as Department Chairman. In 1992, I answered an add for a pediatric radiologist at Loma Linda, because I wanted to have a position where I could teach Radiology. I retired from active practice in 2004 at the rank of Associate Professor. My role at Loma Linda, because of my experience in orthopedic diseases was that of section head for musculoskeletal diseases. During the time that I was at Loma Linda, I became a Fellow of the American College of Radiology and a member of the International Skeletal Society. My career spanned a time of incredible change in Radiology with the advent of computed tomography and later magnetic resonance imaging. Because of the proximity of south Florida to deep sea fishing, that became a lifetime love of mine, and I have enjoyed fishing in Baja California, Hawaii, Australia, New Zealand, and Costa Rica. Throughout my school years prior to college, I studied violin, and was a member of my junior and senior high school orchestras. I love to paint, and have dedicated myself to water colors in the last few years. I love to write, and have written a number of articles on musculoskeletal diseases, but the last year has been consumed with the writing of the Hindman-Webb family story.

When I was recruited by Loma Linda in 1992, I was aware of the many centers of excellence that were part of Loma Linda. I was introduced to a relatively new facility, the Proton Treatment Center, which would become one of its greatest achievements. When I was finally diagnosed with prostate cancer following a long succession of rising PSAs and an earlier negative biopsy, I should have been well positioned to move to proton radiation for the treatment of my tumor. That was not the case. All treatment options initially passed through my urologists, and I had three; one from Loma Linda, one from Templeton, a town close to my retirement home, and a friend of 40 years and Godfather of our oldest child, who is Department Chairman of Urology at a large university medical center. I could have talked to 100 urologists and the answer would have been the same; get the tumor out, and save radiation for another day. I was frightened of the side effects of surgery, most particularly urinary incontinence. Several people were most influential in my final decision to have proton radiation. A former fellow radiology resident and friend of 38 years, had had a trans-perineal radical prostatectomy a year earlier, and he said that if he had it to do over again, he would not have surgery. A close friend and gastroenterologist in my retirement community favored proton therapy over other forms of radiation, because of the ability of protons to give up all their energy at the target, and thus sparing the rectum. My local urologist and I discussed the possibility of pelvic node involvement and the possibility of cutting through tumor at the junction of the prostate and membranous urethra. He thought that the likelihood of cutting across tumor, because of lower quadrant disease was 15-20%, and if that happened, pelvic radiation would be needed. At that instant, I made decision to have proton radiation as the primary and only form of treatment if I would be accepted.

On my first day of treatment I was frightened. I made the three 90 degree turns into the treatment area thinking, this is like Poe's The Cask of Amontillado; I am going to be chained to a treatment table, and never leave the department. Dr. Martell assured me that Loma Linda had never had a patient enter the treatment area and not come out. Then I saw the gantry peaking through tiny windows and a treatment nozzle located at a recessed area suggestive of the entrance of the Holland Tunnel. As I lay in the pod, my thoughts paraphrased the Wizard of Oz, "pay no attention to that monster behind the shield." Quickly my fear changed, first to awe, and then to curiosity and comfort.

Three things have most impressed me during my weeks as a patient. I am in awe of the scientific underpinning of the facility and staff. I am impressed by the staff responsible for the emotion and spiritual health of the patient. They have exemplified the Loma Linda mission statement, to make man whole, better than anything in my experience, including other treatment areas of Loma Linda University Medical Center. Finally, I have been impressed by the intensity, commitment, and intelligence my fellow patients and former patients have brought to the selection of this treatment option as most appropriate for them.

I think that prostate cancer has been a blessing. I have had a very treatable form of malignancy treated with state of the art technology. At the same time, I have learned lessons of advocacy and wholeness that will last for the rest of my life. I will continue to be available to anyone needing understanding and encouragement for proton therapy and life after prostate cancer.

May God bless all of you.

Bernard W. Hindman, M.D.
E-mail: berniehindman@aol.com

Visit www.protonbob.com to read 130 additional testimonials

Appendix C

References

Books

American Cancer Society, *American Cancer Society's Complete Guide to Prostate Cancer*

Centeno, Arthur, Onik, Gary, Kusler, Jack Allen, *Prostate Cancer – A Patient's Guide to Treatment*

Hennenfent M.D., Bradley, *Surviving Prostate Cancer without Surgery*

Kaltenbach, Don, with Tim Richards, *Prostate Cancer, A Survivor's Guide*

Lange, Paul H., and Adamec, Christine, *Prostate Cancer for Dummies*

Lyon Howe, Desiree, *His Prostate and Me*

Marks M.D., Sheldon, *Prostate and Cancer, A Family Guide to Diagnosis, Treatment and Survival.*

Priest, James D., *Beating Prostate Cancer without Surgery*

Ricketts, David, *Eat to Beat Prostate Cancer Cookbook*

Sandage, Stanley, *He Said, 'You Have Prostate Cancer'*

Strum M.D., Stephen and Pogliano, Donna, *A Primer on Prostate Cancer*

Wallner, Kent, *Prostate Cancer – A Non-Surgical Perspective*

Walsh M.D., Patrick, *The Prostate: A Guide for Men and the Women Who Love Them*

Articles:

Clinical Applications of Proton Radiation Treatment at Loma Linda University: Review of a Fifteen-Year Experience, Jerry D. Slater, M.D. Technology in Cancer Research and Treatment, Volume 5, Number 2, April 2006.

Comparison of Conventional-Dose v. High-Dose Conformal Radiation Therapy in Clinically Localized Adenocarcinoma of the Prostate, Anthony Zietman M.D., Jerry d. Slater M.D., Carl Rossi M.D. et. al. Journal of the American Medical Association, Vol.294, No. 10, September 14, 2005

Conformal Proton Beam Radiotherapy of Cancer, Carl J. Rossi, Jr., MD, Department of Radiation Medicine, Loma Linda University Medical Center, Loma Linda, California, March 5, 1996

Considering Radiation for Prostate Cancer, Johns Hopkins Medical Letter. Volume 17, Issue 6, August 2005

Curing Prostate Cancer, Forbes. November 1, 2004

Laparoscopic radical prostatectomy: perioperative complications in an initial and consecutive series of 80 cases, Eur Urol. 2003 Aug;44(2):190-4

Natural history of progression after PSA elevation following radical prostatectomy, Journal of the American Medical Association. 281(17):1591-1597, 1999 C.R. Pound, et al.

Prostate Cancer Tests Might Miss One In Seven Cases, Daily University Science News July 2001

Prostate Health – Early Detection, Informed Choices, Mayo Clinic Health Letter, June 2005.

Prostate-specific antigen doubling times in patients who have failed radical prostatectomy-correlation with histologic characteristics of the primary cancer, Urology. 49:737-742, 1997 R.S. Pruthi, et al.

Proton Therapy for Prostate Cancer – The Initial Loma Linda Experience, Journal of Radiation Oncology, Biology, Physics Vol. 59, No. 2, pp 348-352, 2004

PSA Threshold for Prostate Cancer Misses a 'Significant' Number of Cancers, J Urol 2001;165:757-760

The Patient Proton, LeRoy Butler, PhD, Professor of Organic Chemistry, Norwich University

The Secrets of Long Life, National Geographic, November 2005

The Treatment of Recurrent Prostate Cancer, Communications Newsletter Volume 15, Number 4 Oct. 1999, Charles E. "Snuffy" Myers, M.D.

To Screen or Not to Screen. The Controversy Over Prostate Cancer. Laboratory Medicine V29, No 8.

Appendix D

Helpful Prostate Cancer Websites

American Cancer Society	www.cancer.org
Brotherhood of the Balloon	www.protonbob.com
Don't Fear the Big Dogs	www.dontfearthebigdogs.com
Glossary of Prostate Cancer Terminology	www.phoenix5.org
Latest Prostate Cancer News (PSA Rising)	www.psa-rising.com
Loma Linda Univ. Proton Treatment Center	www.llu.edu/proton
Mayo Clinic Prostate Cancer	www.mayoclinic.com/health/prostate-cancer/DS00043
Memorial Sloan Kettering Prostate Cancer Cure Rate Prediction Tool (Nomogram)	www.mskcc.org/mskcc/html/10088.cfm
National Association for Proton Therapy	www.proton-therapy.org
National Prostate Cancer Coalition	www.fightprostatecancer.org
Patient Insurance advocacy	www.patientadvocate.org
Phoenix 5 Glossary of Terms	www.phoenix5.org/glossary/glossary.html

Prostate Cancer and Proton Treatment	www.prostateproton.com
Prostate Cancer Foundation	www.prostatecancerfoundation.org
Prostate Cancer Meets Proton Beam – A Patient's Experience	www.protons.com
Prostate Cancer Radiation Treatment Sites	www.ecpcp.org
Prostate Cancer Research Institute (PCRI)	www.prostate-cancer.org
Prostate Forum	www.prostateforum.com
Prostate Specific Antigen (PSA)	www.oncolink.org/oncotips/article.cfm?c=5&s=14&ss=21&id=13
Proton vs. Surgery and Conventional Radiation	www.oncolink.org/treatment/article.cfm?c=9&s=70&id=211
The Differences Between Protons and X-Rays	www.oncolink.org/treatment/article.cfm?c=9&s=70&id=210
The History of Proton Therapy	www.oncolink.org/treatment/article.cfm?c=9&s=70&id=209
Proton Beam Therapy Research Giving Back	www.protonresearch.org
Track Your PSA	www.trackyourpsa.com
Us Too-Prostate Cancer Education/Support	www.ustoo.com
You Are Not Alone	www.yananow.net

Helpful Websites (Continued)
Current Functioning
Proton Treatment Centers

Francis H. Burr Proton
Therapy Center
Massachusetts General
Hospital
Began Treating Patients 2002

www.massgeneral.org/cancer/ab
out/providers/radiation/proton

Loma Linda University
Medical Center
Proton Treatment Center
Began Treating Patients 1990

www.llu.edu/proton

MD Anderson Proton Therapy
Center
Began Treating Patients 2006

www.mdanderson.org/care_cent
ers/radiationonco/ptc/

Midwest Proton Therapy
Institute (MPRI)
Began Treating Patients 2004

www.mpri.org

University of Florida Proton
Therapy Institute (Shands
Hospital)
Began Treating Patients 2006

www.floridaproton.org

Appendix E

Premier pathology labs in the U.S.

For Second Opinion on Biopsy Pathology Slides

David Bostwick M.D. M.B.A.   800-214-6628
Bostwick Laboratories, Glen Allen, VA

David Grignon M.D.   313-745-2520
Dept. of Pathology, Wayne State University
Detroit, MI

Dianon Laboratories   800-328-2666
Stratford, CT

Francisco Civantos M.D.   305-325-5587
University of Miami School of Medicine
Miami, FL

John McNeal M.D.   650-725-5534
Department of Urology, Stanford University
Stanford, CA

Jonathan Epstein   410-955-5043
Johns Hopkins Hospital
Baltimore, MD

Jonathan Oppenheimer M.D.   888-868-7522
OUR Lab
Nashville, TN

Appendix F

Medical Insurance Providers That Reimburse for Proton Therapy

The providers listed below have all reportedly reimbursed for proton therapy. This does not necessarily guarantee automatic approval for all. Some of the approvals came after lengthy appeals. Check the entire list, as provider names are listed in several forms.

- AARP
- Aetna
- Aetna US HealthCare
- AFLAC
- Aid Ass'n for Lutherans
- Alberta Blue Cross
- Alberta Government Health Plan
- Amer. Family
- American Association of Lutherans
- American Medical Security
- American National, Galveston
- Anthem BC/BS
- Anthem Blue Cross / Blue Shield of Indiana
- Bankers Life
- Benefit Assistance
- BC/BS
- Blue Cross / Blue Shield of Alabama
- Blue Cross / Blue Shield of California
- Blue Cross / Blue Shield of CO
- BC/BS Federal Employees
- BC/BS of Florida
- BCBS Iowa
- BCBS of Illinois
- Blue Cross of Louisiana
- CARE FIRST Maryland Blue Cross / Blue Shield

- BC/BS of Michigan
- Blue Cross / Blue Shield of Minnesota
- BCBS of Nevada
- BCBS of New Mexico
- Blue Cross / Blue Shield of New York
- BC/BS of North Carolina
- Blue Cross / Blue Shield of Oregon
- BCBS of Western PA
- Blue Cross / Blue Shield of Texas
- Blue Cross/PORAC
- California Care
- CHAMPUS (now TRICARE)
- Christian Fidelity Life Ins. Co.
- CIGNA
- Cityhss
- Continental
- Country Life
- Delta Pilots Medical Plan
- Empire Blue Cross/Blue Shield
- Equitable Life & Casualty
- Firefighters Local
- First Choice
- Freedom Life
- G.I.C. (Unicare)
- GEHA
- German DKV
- GHI
- Golden Rule
- Government Employees Hospital Assoc.
- Government of Ontario CA
- Great West
- Group Health Co-op
- Group Health Co-op of Puget Sound
- Harrington Benefits
- Hartford
- HCF
- Health Net
- Health Partners

- Healthspring
- Heritage Health Plans PPO
- Horizon Blue Cross / Blue Shield
- Humana W. of KY
- Kaiser
- KPS Business Basic
- Lifewise
- Lifewise Health Plan of Washington
- Loma Linda Medical Group
- Mail Handlers
- MDIPA
- Med Care
- Medica
- Medica Choice MN
- Medicaid
- Medi-Cal
- Medical Mutual
- Medical Mutual of Ohio
- Medicare
- Montana Unified School Trust
- Monumental
- Mutual of Omaha
- Nat. Auto. Sprinkler
- National States
- Nationwide
- Nevada Care
- N. Tex Healthcare
- ODS Health Plan
- ODS Of Oregon
- Officers Union
- P.E.R.S. Care
- PacifiCare
- Partners
- PEEHIP of Alabama BC/BS
- PEIA Acordia
- Physicians Mutual
- Primecare for Life
- Pioneer Life

- Premara Blue Cross
- Prudential
- Regence Blue Cross / Blue Shield of Oregon
- Regency Blue Shield
- Rio Grande Employees Hospital Assn.
- Risk Management
- Rocky Mountain HMO
- SAG
- Scott & White Health Plan
- Secure Horizons
- Starmark
- Sterling Option 1
- TRICARE
- Trigon (Now Anthem Blue Cross and Blue Shield)
- TROA Mediplus
- TRS Care
- Tufts HMO
- Unicare
- Uniform (WA state)
- Union Pacific Emp. Health Assoc.
- United American
- United Health Care
- Univera
- UPREHS
- USAA
- Value Health
- Wausaw
- Zurich

To arrange media interviews, personal appearances,

or special assistance the author may be able to provide,

send an e-mail to Bob Marckini at

RMarckini@protonbob.com

~

To order more copies of

You Can Beat Prostate Cancer

by Robert J. Marckini

visit: www.protonbob.com

or send an e-mail to

RMarckini@protonbob.com